Praise for Bright Kids Who Can't Keep Up

"Finally, a book that tackles processing speed head on! After my son was diagnosed with slow processing speed, I began searching for answers. This is the first book that focuses on all the aspects of slow processing speed: home life, school life, and the emotional toll. Just like my son, the children described in this book all want to work hard and do well, but something is blocking them from thriving. The authors guide you to make a consistent, targeted plan to help your child live up to his or her potential. As a teacher, this book is also helping me understand and address learning issues that I often see in the classroom."

—*Sarah R., parent*

"Superb, immensely helpful, authoritative; written with clarity, insight, and pizzazz. Highly recommended."

—*Edward Hallowell, MD, coauthor of*
Driven to Distraction

"If you picture child development as a marathon, life for kids with processing speed issues is more like a steeplechase, with barriers and obstacles that have enormous implications for learning and social and emotional development. This book offers parents an extraordinary gift of knowledge and wisdom to aid in recognizing, understanding, and addressing the challenges of slow processing speed. Drs. Braaten and Willoughby help you accommodate your child's needs and promote essential skills so he or she can thrive."

—*Jerrold F. Rosenbaum, MD, Chief of Psychiatry,*
Massachusetts General Hospital; Stanley Cobb
Professor of Psychiatry, Harvard Medical School

"Parents in our neurodevelopmental clinic often ask, 'If my kid is so smart, why is he so slow?' Finally, there is a book to help parents understand processing speed and its impact on learning and behavior. Drs. Braaten and Willoughby explain the unique way your child engages with the world and discuss ways to overcome challenges, rather than simply offering labels. I will keep a copy of this book on my desk and add it to the short list of parenting books I unconditionally recommend."

—*Sam Goldstein, PhD, Neurology, Learning,*
and Behavior Center, Salt Lake City, Utah

"Drs. Braaten and Willoughby do an exceptional job of deconstructing the complex construct of processing speed. Through examples, articulate explanations of testing results, and clear descriptions of brain processes, this book provides a road map for parents."

—*Timothy E. Wilens, MD, author of* Straight Talk
about Psychiatric Medications for Kids

Bright Kids Who Can't Keep Up

Also available

For General Readers

Straight Talk about Psychological Testing for Kids
Ellen Braaten and Gretchen Felopulos

For Professionals

The Child Clinician's Report-Writing Handbook
Ellen Braaten

Bright Kids
Who Can't Keep Up

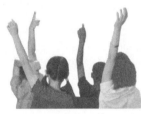

Help Your Child Overcome
Slow Processing Speed
and Succeed
in a Fast-Paced World

Ellen Braaten, PhD
Brian Willoughby, PhD

THE GUILFORD PRESS
New York   London

© 2014 The Guilford Press
A Division of Guilford Publications, Inc.
72 Spring Street, New York, NY 10012
www.guilford.com

Printed in the United States of America

This book is printed on acid-free paper.

Last digit is print number: 9   8   7   6   5   4   3   2

Library of Congress Cataloging-in-Publication data is available from
the publisher.

ISBN 978-1-60918-472-8 (paper) — ISBN 978-1-4625-1549-3 (hard)

For Peter, who has taught me that going at one's
own pace is the only pace worth living

—E. B.

For Nathan, Laurie, Lyle, and Cheryl—
your unwavering support of my education
and career has helped me achieve my personal best

—B. W.

Contents

PART III

Staying Informed

Purchasers can download and print
select practical tools from this book
at *www.guilford.com/braaten3-forms*.

Preface

"My child just had a WISC test, and the examiner said he had very weak processing speed. What does that mean?"

"No matter what I do, my child is slower than any of his peers to get things done. Is there any way to speed him up?"

"My child was diagnosed with ADHD, but she's anything but hyperactive. In fact she's just so slow to get moving on anything. How can that be?"

All of these questions relate to one particular neuropsychological construct: processing speed. As you'll find out in this book, this is a somewhat difficult concept to describe, but its effects, when less than optimal, are more common than most parents realize. Difficulties with processing speed cut across disorders, such as learning disabilities, developmental disorders, and attention problems, and can be quite frustrating for children and their parents. When parents learn that processing speed is a challenge for their child, they often feel relieved that there is an explanation and are eager to know how they can help their child overcome this issue.

As two child psychologists who evaluate hundreds of children each year at the Learning and Emotional Assessment Program (LEAP) at Massachusetts General Hospital and Harvard Medical School, we have found that questions about processing speed are among the most common ones we hear. Fortunately, these questions can be answered because we have a solid base of information from extensive clinical experience, on top of our own research and that of others. The parents we see not only want to understand their child's neurocognitive profile; they want to know how to fix the problems they are living with every day—the pauses as their child tries to take in information, the long time it takes the child to act on instructions, the fact that the child seems to be at the back of every pack, the endless homework sessions. They want to know if their child's symptoms will ever improve and, if not, how to learn to live with a child who functions at a different pace from some or all of the rest of the family.

This book is an attempt to anticipate and answer the questions you may have when you find that your child has a slow processing speed. Although we don't have answers to every question, we do supply the facts about what processing speed is, how it affects family and social relationships, and how it impacts school performance. We provide guidelines for how to cope with and treat this issue. There's a lot you can do to compensate for your child's processing speed to make sure your child succeeds—at home, at school, in the social world—and remains happy and endowed with healthy self-esteem. Above all, we hope you will realize that your child's issues are not unique and that your situation is far from hopeless.

Acknowledgments

Those of you who have been a part of our lives over the 3 years that it took us to write this book have appreciated the irony of taking 2 years too long to write a book about how to make kids do things faster. In fact, *appreciate* may be the wrong word to describe how you feel about us, although it is the best way for us to describe how we feel about you. We relied on many people over the course of this project, most specifically our families, who at times were worried we were spending more time talking about why we weren't finished with the book than actually writing the book. You know who you are, and you're probably happier than we are that we are done.

Our editors at The Guilford Press, Kitty Moore and Chris Benton, were not just outstanding at editing the manuscript and helping us develop the topic; they also were patient with us as we took our time getting the ideas down on paper. When we first discussed this topic with Kitty, it was hard to describe to her why the book needed to be written, yet Kitty trusted us when we said that this is an issue that parents struggle with on a daily basis. She and Chris then helped us articulate the issues and the solutions behind the struggles. A writer could not find two better friends, mentors, critics, and supporters. We benefited considerably from their wisdom, insight, and sense of humor.

We have to give a big thank you to our colleagues at LEAP. There is not a better group of people anywhere, and each and every staff person, post-doc, and intern who has graced the halls of LEAP has influenced our thinking in this book. A particular thanks goes to Darlene Maggio, who keeps our lives sane and who helped us with small and large details with this project. We'd be lost without you.

We thank our family and friends who supported us throughout this process. And to James Olofson, who helped with the illustrations and graphics—we can't thank you enough for all of your time. Further, Hannah Braaten deserves a very special thank you for being our trusted first reader and then finally saying, "You just need to get it done" when, well, it was time to just get it done. She is the best daughter—ever.

Lastly, the muses behind this book are the parents and children we see every day. You have educated us and inspired us. We hope that in reading this book you realize that you are not alone.

PART I

Understanding Processing Speed

"If My Kid Is So Smart, Why Is He So Slow?"

"I can see why everyone is so frustrated with Dennis, because I'm frustrated with him too! He can't get *anything* done on time. Whether it's his homework, putting on his shoes, or taking down a phone message, he *can't* get it done! If I didn't know him so well, I'd think he just didn't care, but I know he does. In fact, he cares a lot. He just doesn't know how to get motivated or get started. His dad thinks he's just lazy, and I have to admit it does seem like that, but I know he would do things faster if he could. He has great ideas and will talk about how excited he is about writing a paper for his history class, but then when it comes time to actually *do* it, he just sits there, seemingly paralyzed with fear—or maybe just daydreaming—I don't know! If he didn't care about the work, he wouldn't be so excited about the topic, right? I try to help him get started by telling him to copy down some ideas on notecards, but it takes him forever to find the information in the book and even longer to just copy it down. It seems he's been like this since he was born. Even in first grade, when he had to just copy—only copy—his spelling words, it would take him 10 times as long as it should have. His father thinks he's lazy, his teachers think he just doesn't care, and I'm spending my life yelling at him to get things done. How did we get into this mess?"

Some kids are naturally fast. They run, talk, draw, and do all sorts of things at a rate that seems appropriate for their age. Other kids don't, or perhaps it would be fairer to say they can't. These are kids who may have what are called *processing speed deficits*. *Information processing speed* is a term that is frequently used in the field of neuropsychology and is used increasingly in the fields of education and child development. As you'll discover in the next few chapters, it is a term that refers to a complex process and so is defined and measured in many ways. It also can't be understood in isolation from other areas of thinking, such as language, memory, or attention.

In general, though, processing speed involves one or more of the following functions: the amount of time it takes to *perceive information* (this can be through any of the senses, but usually through the visual and auditory channels), *process information,* and/or *formulate or enact a response.* Another way to define processing speed is to say it's *the time required to perform an intellectual task* or *the amount of work that can be completed with a certain period of time.* Even more simply, processing speed could be defined as *how long it takes to get stuff done.*

Because we place such a high value on doing things quickly in our culture, it can be difficult to live with a nervous system that needs more time to process information. Kids and adults who are slower at these types of processing tasks are sometimes assumed to be lacking in intelligence, but this really isn't the case. However, processing speed does interact with other areas of cognitive functioning by negatively impacting the ability to quickly come up with an answer, retrieve information from long-term memory, and remember what you're supposed to be doing at a given time. In other words, it's possible that someone with slow processing speed will, as a result, be impaired in other areas of thinking and may even score lower on tests of intelligence (more about this area in the next chapter), but this isn't necessarily the case, since being cognitively compromised in one area isn't the same as being less intelligent overall.

For example, Dennis was actually a very intelligent kid, with a Verbal IQ in the 90th percentile of kids his age, even though his actions and thought processes seemed so slow. Dennis's slow output seems to be disconnected from his natural intellect, which creates the assumption that he's just not capable of completing even simple homework tasks such as copying his weekly spelling words.

Dennis's family has endured countless episodes where his lack of productivity has made their daily life a constant battleground. Many of the instances at home involve homework and chore completion. Often Dennis will just shrug his shoulders when he has disappointed his parents by not doing something they've asked him to do, but other times he reacts angrily and tells them they just don't "get it." "You think I can do this, but I can't!" is a frequent retort.

One mental health professional told Dennis's parents that he possibly had something called oppositional defiant disorder; another said he exhibited symptoms of attention-deficit/hyperactivity disorder (ADHD), and still another said to just "let it go" because he was just "being a boy." Dennis's teacher and the school psychologist thought it could be a "processing problem," but they never explained what that meant or how they had come to that conclusion.

Dennis's parents didn't think any of these labels or explanations fit perfectly or captured the upheaval, turmoil, and trauma created by Dennis's inability to complete work in a timely fashion. His inability to finish his homework required constant vigilance and enormous energy from his parents. The effort his parents spent trying to help him get things done created even more resentment from his siblings. His parents were constantly fighting over how to handle his difficulties. They felt angry, frustrated, overwhelmed, worn out, and hopeless—and they had no idea what to do or where to turn.

"So How Do I Know That My Child Has a Slow Processing Speed?"

Perhaps you picked up this book because you have a child like Dennis, or perhaps the idea of a child being smart but unable to keep up resonated with you. Perhaps you've sought help from mental health or school professionals, some of whom might have advised making sure your child gets enough sleep, eats a better breakfast, "comes to school ready to learn," or that you be more consistent in managing your child's behavior. Perhaps you've tried all of those suggestions. Perhaps you didn't need to because you knew it wasn't just a sleep or motivational issue but something else about your child's learning or cognitive style that had yet to be explained.

True processing speed deficits should be evaluated through a formal assessment by a professional such as a psychologist, as they are usually an indication of another underlying problem, the most common being attention problems. A diagnosis of the inattentive subtype of ADHD often comes with slow processing speed, although that's not always the case.

The second largest category of children with processing speed deficits are those with learning disabilities, such as dyslexia, nonverbal learning disabilities, language-based learning disabilities, and autism spectrum disorders (including pervasive developmental disorder and Asperger syndrome). Although processing speed deficits are not the underlying cause of the learning disability, many children with learning and developmental issues exhibit processing speed deficits as part of their cognitive profile.

Other children who may suffer from more transient processing speed deficits are those with psychological issues such as depression, anxiety, or psychosocial stressors (such as the loss of a parent). Children in this category may show processing speed problems only when their symptoms of depression are severe enough that they can't get things done or when they are so anxious that their perfectionistic tendencies make them complete work extremely slowly.

A final category of children are those who don't fall into any of these categories, but who perform poorly on all (or at least most) timed tests as compared to untimed tests. This category of children has in the past sometimes been diagnosed with something called a "learning disorder, not otherwise specified (processing speed deficits)." More recent terminology may refer to it as a learning disability with a specific impairment in reading, writing, or math fluency. In most of these cases, the diagnosis has been made by a licensed professional, most likely a psychologist, after formal testing has been completed. If your child has not had a thorough evaluation, consider the pros and cons of pursuing an evaluation that are explored in Chapter 2.

The entire first section of this book is devoted to helping you understand the importance of processing speed, what it is, and how it affects your and your child's lives. What we've found is that dealing more effectively with processing speed deficits first and foremost requires an understanding of what it is. Once you understand that it isn't always in your child's control to be the quickest one in the family—and once you have a better sense as to *why* your child behaves as she does—the strategies for helping her become clearer. In some cases, just *understanding* your child's deficits can lead to improvements in your child's life (particularly in her relationship with you) even before you try some of the strategies outlined in this book.

The middle section of the book helps you think about how processing speed deficits specifically impact your child in particular environments and what you can do to help. We'll also discuss the unfortunate emotional toll this deficit takes on kids who can't keep up and how to lessen the impact of anxiety, depression, and low self-esteem often caused by slow processing speed. In the third section, we bring it all together and show what a full evaluation looks like, using a few typical examples, and what types of recommendations might flow from a thorough assessment. We also tell you where to go for more information from websites and books that can fill in the gaps. Throughout the book you'll read about strategies that have been helpful to many of the children, families, and teachers with whom we've worked over the years.

Although processing speed may vary as a function of a child's age and underlying issue, most cases do share some common threads that contribute to difficulties at school and home, such as slow reading and writing, slow response to requests or questions (even those as simple as "What do you want for breakfast?"), poor memory recall, and slow completion of work. When these issues go untreated, it can sometimes lead a child to avoid homework or, in extreme cases, avoid school altogether. These children may appear unmotivated, sluggish, apathetic, and with low energy. Even getting started on tasks is difficult for them. When they have trouble sustaining attention at school or in meetings, they may drift into daydreams, stare blankly into space, or even sleep. They may become fidgety, tapping their pencil or foot, play with their hair or the paper clip on their desk, or ask to go to the bathroom frequently. These types of "coping mechanisms" often lead teachers to think these student don't care, when actually they have "checked out" because the pace of the environment was too quick for them to access.

Processing Speed in Daily Life

In everyday life, there is a cost to processing everything more slowly. Some jobs demand a fast pace. In fact, it would be impossible to perform certain jobs without that quick rate of response. Emergency room doctors, jet pilots, and air traffic controllers, among dozens of other careers, place a high priority on the ability to react to information and quickly perform tasks.

Though it might not be obvious, these sorts of skills are important in school as well. From being asked to complete "1-minute math worksheets" in second grade, to the ability to move between classes and rooms in middle and high school (while remembering to get the appropriate books and assignments from a locker in a 4-minute transition period), the ability to do things quickly is highly related to a child's success in school. Some examples of the types of problems that children with slow processing speed experience include:

- Difficulty processing spoken information fluently or automatically:
  - Problems listening to a lecture and taking in all the material presented
  - Remembering and following simple directions from a teacher
  - Listening and understanding verbal information presented in class from fellow students
- Problems writing information down on paper:
  - Writing an assignment in a notebook
  - Finishing an exam
- Slower reading fluency skills:
  - Having difficulty reading a certain passage in a given period of time during class time or during exams
  - Difficulty finishing large reading assignments
- Trouble sustaining attention to a task, not necessarily because the child has attention problems, but because the information is coming at her so quickly that her attention is "lost"
- Difficulty understanding complex directions, particularly those that are given quickly
- Trouble retrieving information quickly from long-term memory. This becomes problematic when a child is called on in class and can't answer the question quickly enough—even though he knows the answer!
- Problems finishing almost anything (tests, assignments, activities) in an allotted period of time
- Problems with social interactions because the "social scene" moves too quickly to process (includes not just verbal information but nonverbal information that has to be processed quickly).

In addition to problems at school, slow processing speed can make life difficult for a family. When there is one person in a family who takes *forever* to do something, the rest of the family suffers.

Take the case of James, a 10-year-old boy with ADHD and extremely slow processing speed, who took three times longer than his 12-year-old sister, Jenny, to complete pretty much any daily task. From the moment James woke up in the morning, he couldn't keep up. It took him 10 minutes to find his way to the bathroom, even longer to pick out what to wear, and it often took him so long to figure out what to have for breakfast that he left for school without eating anything. Jenny, on the other hand, was quick to dress and was ready for the school bus on time, although her mornings were punctuated by her mother shouting, "James, if you don't get down here, I'm going to scream!"

Jenny was embarrassed that the bus had to wait for her brother nearly every morning. Things were worse after school, when James couldn't get his homework done without constant pleading and coaxing from one of his parents. Dinnertime took forever because James was slow to get to the table, slow to decide what he wanted to eat, and slow to actually eat his food. Jenny's relationship with her brother suffered, and she often found herself angry about these disruptions. Not surprisingly, James's parents found themselves frustrated and sad that their family life was miserable at times because they were always yelling at James or bribing him to hurry up.

James's story is very typical for children with slow processing speed. Although he demonstrated many of the characteristics mentioned above in school, his problems at home were also quite significant. Some of the more common problems that children with slow processing speed experience at home include:

- Slowness in getting out of bed in the morning and getting ready for the day

- Difficulty getting ready for bed at night, as well as difficulty falling asleep—yes, these kids are even slow to fall asleep!

- Trouble making up their minds about everyday tasks such as what they are going to wear or what they want for breakfast

- Slow at eating to an extent that mealtimes seem to take forever or their food is cold before they are finished

- Slow to complete simple tasks such as brushing their teeth or taking a shower

- Problems starting tasks such as homework

- Problems completing homework in a reasonable amount of time

- Difficulty completing chores, even simple chores like taking out the trash

- Slowness in remembering information about family matters, such as quickly remembering the name of a relative they haven't seen in a while, or remembering that the family is going on vacation next week. This can lead family members to think the child is "in his own world" or worse, that she "just doesn't care about anyone but herself."

For example, James had trouble fully taking in the following when his mom said one Saturday, "Today we're going to see the new *Harry Potter* movie at the mall, but first I need to stop at the dry cleaner's and then take you to get new shoes because we're going to Aunt Dottie's wedding next week. And, maybe we'll get you a new shirt too, while we're at it, and then when we're done with the movie, we can get ice cream." James's mom was talking quickly as she was cleaning up the breakfast dishes. So when she said, "Go get ready so we can go to the movies," James replied, "What movie? I thought you were taking me out for ice cream right now." Needless to say, his mother was aggravated because he "wasn't listening," when actually he was listening but it was too much information for him to process in the amount of time needed.

Types of Processing Speed

Processing speed isn't a one-dimensional concept. It's not just about how fast we see, or how fast we write, or how fast we can process what we've heard. It's really a combination of all of those factors. In fact, processing speed deficits can be observed in *visual processing, verbal processing,* and *motor speed.* Problems in one or more of these areas can manifest in problems with *academic fluency* and *general difficulties.* However, it is rare to be slow at *all* of the above. For example, a child with a language-based learning disability may be quite slow to interpret spoken language, but she might be very quick on the soccer field because she has quicker visual processing abilities. In that case, her problems with auditory processing speed may get in the way of her athletic skills when she is required to put into practice the coach's directions quickly. In another example, a child might understand spoken language at an age-appropriate pace, but she may not have the motor speed to put her thoughts on paper at a pace that is typical of her peers. While speed is central to all of these processing abilities, they do, of course, vary considerably in how they are manifested in daily life and on more formal measures of processing speed.

VISUAL PROCESSING

Visual processing relates to how quickly our eyes perceive information and relay it to the brain. In its simplest form, it can be measured as to how quickly our eyes dilate to light or how quickly we respond to a visual stimulus. It's related to almost anything we do. Drivers with slower visual processing have slower visual reaction times and get into more accidents. Studies have shown that individuals with slower visual processing have difficulties with tasks such as looking up phone numbers, reading directions, counting out change, and finding an item on a crowded shelf.

VERBAL PROCESSING

Verbal processing, not surprisingly, relates to how quickly we hear a stimulus and react to it. "Reacting" may include a simple motor reaction (such as expressive surprise or moving when something is startling) or more complex problem solving such as making meaning from what someone has said and then reacting to it by providing a cogent verbal response. Research has shown that problems with verbal processing speed are related to problems with nearly all aspects of verbal memory and comprehending instructions.

MOTOR SPEED

Within the field that studies processing speed, *motor speed* generally relates to fine motor agility, such as how fast we can copy something or put pegs in a board, rather than to how fast someone can run, for example. This is one of the areas of processing speed that's been studied the most, primarily because it's relatively easy to study. Some methods of testing processing speed include timed tests that measure the speed at which someone can place pegs in a grooved board (motor speed), copy a series of numbers (visual and motor processing speed), or read a paragraph (visual and verbal speed processing). In all of these examples, visual processing plays a role in how quickly these tasks can be completed. Thus, when we talk about *academic fluency*, such as how quickly it takes to complete a math worksheet, write a paragraph, or copy something from a blackboard, we're really talking about a complex interaction of visual and motor skills (often referred to as *visual–motor* skills). Depending on the task, verbal processing may also play a role. For example, taking notes in class depends on a person's ability to quickly *hear and understand* what someone is saying, *visually process* what a teacher has written on the chalkboard, and use *motor speed* in writing the information in a notebook.

EFFECTS ON GENERAL FUNCTIONING

Processing speed deficits in one or more areas often lead to deficits in *general areas of functioning*. It can mean that a child needs more time to complete many—if not most—tasks. A child may often look confused or appear absentminded because he is unable to process information at the rate it's being delivered. Some children may actually avoid engaging in difficult tasks altogether or not get started on new tasks because they are aware they cannot get the job done in the amount of time allotted, and therefore feel defeated before they even begin. Conversely some kids cope with these deficits by rushing through their work; they may finish a test quickly and turn it in even though they haven't answered each question thoroughly. The work might not be completed correctly, but the student feels a sense of accomplishment because he wasn't the last one done.

Maturation of Processing Speed during Childhood (or, "Will My Kid Ever Get Any Faster?")

The million-dollar question that we get asked almost on a daily basis is "Will this ever get better?" It is one of the toughest questions to answer, and more about this will be said in Chapter 3 (which explores the science of processing speed). The short answer is *yes*. Nearly every child will be faster at age 10 than she was at age 5—and even faster at age 15. The problem is that everyone else is getting faster too, and processing speed is relative. So even though a child is faster than she was before, it's possible (or even likely) that she'll still be slower when compared to peers. However, a child's processing speed does change dramatically over time, and a number of different factors contribute to these changes.

First, the changes are likely related to the impact of practice and experience. Since young children are relatively inexperienced at nearly all tasks (even simple ones like brushing their teeth and deciding what to wear), their lack of experience leads to slower processing. Research on processing speed has shown that the more times someone repeats a task, the more automatic—and thus quicker—the response becomes. This is why even kids with slow processing speed are quicker than their parents on tasks such as video games and texting on a cell phone.

Second, the speed increases are also due to structural changes to the brain that happen naturally as it develops during childhood. So, for example, just as changes in computers have "grown" over the years to produce faster central processing, so does growth in the brain result in faster cognitive processing times. These changes include more connections in the central nervous system, brain growth, and changes in something called *myelination*. The *myelin sheath* is a layer of fatty cells that insulates the brain's nerve cells and helps speed the brain's impulses. Just as electrical current needs to be insulated, so do the brain's electrical impulses. During childhood, that insulation develops (this is the process of *myelination*), and it allows the brain to work more efficiently and quickly because the electrical impulses that form the base of the functioning of the brain can travel faster and more effectively—all of which culminates in the ability to literally *think faster.*

These two factors—experience and brain growth—are crucial in increasing processing speed during the childhood and adolescent years. Do most kids speed up? With the exception of children who have significant brain trauma, nearly every child will become faster at most things. The problem is that you, as a parent, might not reap the benefits as the process continues into young adulthood. By the time your child is ready to go to college, he will probably be ready to make up his mind about what to have for breakfast quickly enough to get to class, though he might still be the last one in the family out the door. Soon after that, he'll be off to college or a job and those maturing—and faster—processing speed skills won't be as apparent to his parents as they will to his roommates, professors, or employers.

As the graph on the next page shows, very often the gap with peers never shrinks. In other words, although your child will be faster than he was several years ago, she'll likely never be *faster than her peers.* The key to dealing with this issue is explored later in the book, but suffice it to say here that in adult life deficits in processing are often not a problem because we generally choose vocations and avocations that are well suited to us. For example, a child with a slower processing speed who also has superior ver-

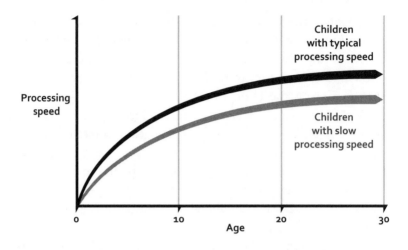

bal skills might be better off as a philosophy professor than a trial lawyer. Although this is a gross generalization to illustrate a point, the issue going forward in life is to keep expectations for growth realistic while maximizing the child's potential. Not every career demands quickness—in fact, for some careers it is a hindrance. Knowing what to expect is key—but more about that in future chapters.

A Quick Assessment of Processing Speed

If you're reading this book, you likely already suspect that your child has slow processing speed. Perhaps she has had formal testing that indicated a deficit, or perhaps you just *know* that your child's natural pace is slower than that of her peers. In the next chapter, we'll talk about formally assessing processing speed, but as an informal assessment, the checklist on pages 17–18 is a good guide. The items on the checklist are broken down into specific areas:

1. Verbal Processing (that is, "Listening")
2. Visual Processing
3. Motoric Processing

The Processing Speed Checklist for Parents

Does your child exhibit problems in the following areas?

1. Verbal Processing

- ❑ Appears not to listen to others
- ❑ Doesn't seem to understand directions
- ❑ Can't seem to follow instructions
- ❑ Becomes overwhelmed with too much verbal information
- ❑ Needs more time to answer questions
- ❑ Even when he knows the right answer, is hesitant to give it
- ❑ Answers questions with short responses
- ❑ Does not participate in class discussions
- ❑ Has trouble retrieving factual information from memory
- ❑ Can't keep up with the pace of lectures
- ❑ Makes grammatical errors in writing
- ❑ Has problems sustaining focused attention during social activities
- ❑ Needs additional time to respond in conversations

2. Visual Processing

- ❑ Doesn't pay close attention to details
- ❑ Has difficulty proofreading work
- ❑ Makes careless errors
- ❑ Doesn't grasp the subtle, visual cues of social relationships
- ❑ Stares off into space instead
- ❑ Neglects to look at important visual information
- ❑ Omits phrases or words in writing

3. Motoric Processing

- ❑ Seems tired, even after a good night's sleep
- ❑ Seems lazy or unmotivated

(cont.)

❏ Moves slowly on fine motor (for example, writing) or gross motor (for example, catching a ball) tasks

❏ Is reluctant to start tasks

❏ Can *do* the assignments, but not in the time allotted

❏ Is slow at the physical aspects of writing

4. *Academic Processing*

❏ Is a slow reader

❏ Is slow to recall basic math facts (for example, times tables)

❏ Has difficulty taking notes in class

❏ Has trouble formulating and expressing ideas in writing

❏ Exhibits inconsistent academic performance

❏ Lacks fluency when reading aloud

❏ Becomes distracted during academic tasks

❏ Makes punctuation and capitalization errors

❏ Makes spelling errors in writing, despite otherwise being a good speller

5. *General Problems with Processing Speed*

❏ Often looks confused

❏ Frequently seems absentminded

❏ Lacks persistence in completing any type of task

❏ Avoids tasks that require sustained attention or focus

❏ Generally seems to be "slow" much of the time

❏ Needs extra time to complete tasks

❏ Forgets information that he learned just yesterday

❏ Frequently responds, "What?"

❏ Starts out strong but then wanders off-task or "tunes out"

❏ Impulsively rushes through tasks

❏ Is hesitant to participate in social situations or conversations

4. Academic Processing
5. General Problems with Processing Speed

Record your answers here to compare with scores on a similar checklist in Chapter 4. In that chapter, which discusses how parents and kids "fit" in terms of their processing speed, you'll get a chance to rate yourself in these areas. It might also be useful to complete the checklist below for *all* of the children in your family, so that you can get a sense of the match between the siblings. If you'd like to do that, feel free to photocopy the checklist or download and print extra copies from *www.guilford.com/braaten3-forms*.

You might find that your child exhibits problems in only a couple of areas or in most areas. The child might vary in how frequently and pervasively she exhibits these problems. Overall, though, as you might have guessed, more "yes" responses are indicative of more significant problems with processing speed.

What We <u>Don't</u> Know about Processing Speed Is More Than What We <u>Do</u> Know

Don't let this statement discourage you. Processing speed has become an increasingly important topic in the field of child development and child psychology; however, we know less about it than we do about almost any other area of cognition—but that doesn't mean we don't know anything about it. Processing speed is a multidimensional variable; it is complex and it is yet to be determined how best to define and measure it. Although we know it has an effect on social, emotional, and academic functioning, we don't yet know *all* that we should to assess it and treat it fully. That being said, we do have some ideas on how to best compensate and remediate impairments in this area. Researchers have started to understand how processing speed is related to other areas of brain functioning, what the possible causes of difficulties are, and how other disorders such as ADHD and learning disabilities contribute to weaknesses in processing speed.

If you are a parent of a child who is frequently described as *always behind, never able to keep up,* this book may restore some optimism to your family and help you feel that you can cope with these difficulties more confidently and competently because you understand them better. If you are reading this book because you have a niece, nephew, or grandchild with these issues, or if you're a teacher or therapist, our hope is that this book will provide the knowledge you need. Although there is no magic bullet that will solve a child's deficits, we do highlight the steps to take to help your child reach his full potential. There is good reason for hope because this is a new and exciting field in the area of cognitive research, and more is being discovered every day.

two

"My Child Doesn't Seem to Be Able to Keep Up . . . Now What Do I Do?"

Parents often feel helpless when their child has a problem and they have no idea how to make things better. If your child seems unable to keep up adequately with his peers, each day brings new challenges and frustrations for him and new worries and fears for you.

Take the case of Sam, who was an absolutely delightful baby and toddler who never gave his parents a bit of trouble. His mother was thrilled that Sam was very different from his older brother, who was always "getting into everything." In fact, Sam never got into anything. He sat quietly watching the world go by from his high chair or stroller. The pace at which he moved was not nearly as quick as that of the other children on the playground, but his parents thought it was refreshing, and other parents described him as a well-behaved and "calm" toddler.

Once he arrived at preschool, things changed for Sam. Instead of being described as "calm," his teacher described him as "having trouble getting with the program." He was the last one off the playground, the last one to finish his snack, and he seemed hesitant to join in group activities. His parents were concerned, but nearly everyone they talked to (including his teacher) said, "Give him time; he'll grow out of it."

Unfortunately, school—and even daily life—continued to present challenges to Sam. By first grade, his teacher asked if his parents had thought about "having him tested." Sam's parents had no idea what that meant, and the teacher had trouble putting into words why it was important and how it could be helpful. It seemed that everyone had trouble describing exactly what was causing Sam to have such a hard time keeping up. His first-grade teacher thought Sam might have ADHD, his second-grade teacher thought it could be a learning disability, and his third-grade teacher said, "If he doesn't get some help, we might be talking about retention." At that point—and after many sleepless nights—his parents decided they had to do *something*. The problem was that they didn't know exactly what it was they needed to *do*.

They started seeking other people's advice when Sam was in third grade. His teacher said, "Sign these papers so that the school can test him. We'll figure out what the problem is and maybe put him on an IEP." Sam's best friend's mother said, "The school wanted to test my child, but I said, 'no way' and I took my child to Dr. X, who diagnosed him with a learning disability." Sam's pediatrician said, "Maybe it'd be a good idea to have a neuropsychological evaluation. Let me get you the name of a neuropsychologist who can help." Finally, a neighbor added her advice by saying, "You just have to apply more discipline. You need to get him into therapy so he learns how to listen."

His parents were lost. Terms such as *IEP, learning disability*, and *neuropsychologist* scared them. What did these things mean? Could they possibly be more harmful than helpful? What if Sam *did* have a *learning disability*? Would that mean he would be labeled as unable to learn? Would that label have long-lasting consequences for him? They had never even heard the term *neuropsychologist*, but it sounded serious. Did this mean there was something wrong with Sam's brain and his pediatrician was afraid to tell them? Or could it be that pursuing one or more of these options was the key to getting Sam back on track?

The Pros and Cons of Formal Assessments

One thing that should be clear from hearing Sam's story is that his parents have options. Options are good—and if you're struggling with concerns about your child's ability to process information quickly, but no one has identified the problem, you've got a number of *really good* options. All of the choices presented by various professionals and laypeople to Sam's parents could be useful, and each has its pros and cons.

You too may have found that various people have given you their input about what to do. You may feel not just confused about the options but also a little hurt or embarrassed when you're trying your best to be a good parent. Our advice is to look at each option critically, regardless of how the option was presented to you. Don't automatically discard a choice just because the way someone said it was insensitive.

If your sister-in-law snapped at the last family reunion, "You know, you should really have that kid see a shrink," it doesn't mean the option couldn't be helpful (though she never needs to know you took her advice!). We've seen parents not pursue evaluations just because they were hurt that someone (a teacher, a pediatrician, a well-meaning relative) brought up the issue of testing or seeing a psychologist in a way that seemed tactless or inconsiderate, when really it was well meaning but poorly stated or (worse) said at the family Christmas party or in front of other parents at the afterschool pickup line.

Testing through the school or privately—or even just getting a one-time consultation with a psychologist—are options that can help you determine how best to help your child, and this information may ultimately help you sleep better at night. So, what are the most common options a parent considers, and what are the pros and cons of each? Pursuing an *evaluation through the school system*, pursuing an *evaluation outside of the school system, getting a briefer consultation* (without pursuing testing), and *waiting and seeing* are all valid alternatives. Let's see how Sam and his parents dealt with the pros and cons of each.

HAVING YOUR CHILD EVALUATED THROUGH THE SCHOOL SYSTEM

When Sam's parents decided to have him evaluated in third grade, they initially decided to pursue an evaluation through the school system. This route had its advantages. First, the evaluation would be done at no cost to them. The school tested Sam using standardized tests (more about this later) that assessed his cognition (or thinking), language, and processing skills. The school's evaluation pinpointed his areas of weakness.

A second advantage of having the school perform the evaluation was that the people who did the assessment were the same people who were going to be involved in Sam's treatment. For the school to do the evaluation, Sam's parents had to sign some forms consenting for the evaluation to be completed at school. It's a legal requirement that schools obtain parental permission before performing this kind of assessment, so if you're thinking about having an evaluation through the school, you'll be given paperwork that outlines the kinds of tests the evaluator is planning to use. You'll need to sign off on the evaluation, and you should read this consent form carefully: You can agree to some parts of the evaluation and not to others. For example, in Sam's case, his parents agreed for the school to do all of the evaluation they suggested with the exception of the speech and language portion, which they opted to have done through a private speech and language therapist who had been referred to them by Sam's pediatrician. They hadn't heard good things about the speech and language therapist at Sam's school and wanted a second opinion.

Sam's parents were pleased with the services (such as academic tutoring) and accommodations (such as extra time on tests) that the school decided to provide after completing the testing. However, they were left feeling a little lost about what was causing the problem. The school referred to "the problem" as a "processing deficit," and they didn't know what that meant. They were experiencing one of the *cons* of receiving an evaluation through the school system; that is, a school evaluation rarely ever results in a diagnosis such as "ADHD" or "reading disability."

In fact, the purpose of a school evaluation isn't to provide a diagnosis for a child's difficulties, but to describe the deficits in enough detail so that remediations and accommodations can be put into place at school. You shouldn't expect a diagnosis or feel cheated that you didn't get one from the school. You also shouldn't expect them to have time to explain what every score on each test means, which is another downside of school testing. We've had parents ask us why the school didn't tell them that their child met criteria for a specific diagnosis. Our answer is simply that it isn't the school's job. However, many times, following a school evaluation, the evaluators, teachers, or administrators will suggest getting a private evaluation or a consultation because they suspect there is something that should be specifically diagnosed.

GETTING AN EVALUATION OUTSIDE THE SCHOOL SYSTEM

By the fifth grade, this is exactly what Sam's team of school specialists suggested to his parents. They had suspected that Sam might have ADHD and that it might be the underlying cause of his processing speed deficits—but they suggested that this possibility be evaluated by an independent psychologist. Sam's parents took their suggestion and had him evaluated by a pediatric

Individually administered tests are used in both school and independent evaluations. These tests are administered one-on-one between the evaluator and your child. The evaluator will ask the child questions, have her complete puzzles, or read aloud. The evaluator will watch closely not only *what* your child says or does but also *how* she does it. These types of tests are very different from the SAT or other tests that are administered in groups. Thus, it's important to choose the evaluator carefully because the rapport between your child and the evaluator can affect the overall experience of the evaluation.

neuropsychologist—a child psychologist who specializes in the assessment of children with learning, developmental, and cognitive disorders. A neuropsychologist uses *individually administered* standardized tests to determine how a person's brain functioning relates to his behavior.

There were some pros to getting Sam evaluated by a private neuropsychologist. First, based on the evidence, the neuropsychologist did diagnose him with ADHD, inattentive subtype, a type of ADHD in which inattention (as opposed to hyperactivity or impulsivity) is the primary symptom. Instead of feeling resentful that their child was being labeled, they were relieved that they finally understood the root of Sam's difficulties. Another pro of the evaluation was that the psychologist spent time reviewing the test results in detail, and Sam's parents finally understood what the numbers and test scores in the reports meant. In contrast to the school's feedback, the evaluator was able to discuss how Sam's profile affected his family life, including his at-times difficult relationship with his brother. She spent time talking to them about their fears for Sam in the future and was available, as needed, by phone when they had further questions.

Unfortunately, the evaluation was not covered by insurance (a frequent con of a private evaluation) and was expensive. However, an important pro of the private evaluation is that private evaluators can often liaise with the child's teachers and with school

As stated in Chapter 1, it's important to remember that *processing speed deficits most often occur in the context of another issue,* such as ADHD, a learning disability, or a developmental disorder. If you're worried that your child is frequently failing to keep up, it might be the sign of a more specific problem that needs further exploration. This is probably the biggest pro to seeking a more formal evaluation: In the course of evaluating processing speed, the evaluator may uncover some other important areas of functioning that are in need of remediation.

administrators. Sam's parents were grateful that his psychologist participated in a conference call with his school in which his teacher, the evaluating psychologist, the special education director, and the guidance counselor could devise a strategy together.

GETTING A BRIEFER CONSULTATION

Were these two routes (school and independent evaluations) the only ones available to Sam and his family? No, there were a couple of other things they could have done. One option would have been to seek a briefer consultation from a professional such as a licensed psychologist. Had Sam's family pursued this option in first grade, the psychologist may have provided his parents with suggestions on how to manage his behaviors at home and how to work best with his teacher to address his difficulties at school. She may have recommended that Sam attend therapy to learn to manage his behavior more appropriately. She may also have suggested further testing and provided the parents with the names of qualified evaluators. Any of these options may have been appropriate at the time.

TAKING THE "WAIT-AND-SEE" APPROACH

Another option (and one that Sam's parents "pursued" for a number of years) is the wait-and-see approach. There's nothing wrong with waiting, and in fact Sam's parents waited until he was in third grade before getting answers to their questions. One reason there's nothing wrong with waiting is that some children actually do outgrow their difficulties (slow processing speed being only one of dozens of difficulties children can experience). A second reason is that parents aren't always quite ready to deal with the issues that might need to be addressed. Sometimes they're scared about what might come to light. This is understandable, but most parents feel better once a potential problem has been identified.

If you choose a wait-and-see approach, our advice would be to participate actively in the problem-solving process while you wait and see. Don't just ignore the issue—*watch* and *seek informa-*

tion. *Watch* to see if your child's difficulties are getting worse—if so, it's probably a good idea to move in the direction of a more formal assessment. At the same time, *seek information* from people you trust. This might mean turning to your child's teacher, pediatrician, or grandparent. If they're all saying "Don't worry yet," then waiting might not be a bad option. However, if your child has a fabulous teacher who has been teaching for 20 years and she says, "I've never had a kid in my class who takes as long to get things done as your Johnny does," then you might want to consider seeking help sooner rather than later.

One word of advice about waiting: After over 30 years of combined experience evaluating children and adolescents, we've never yet had a parent who has said to either of us, "I wish I'd waited a year or two to get my child evaluated." In fact, rarely does a week go by when we don't hear, "Why didn't I do this sooner?" We've seen many Sams after they've experienced year after year of perceived failures at school, and who, by age 16, are frequently depressed or angry or worse—completely fed up with the learning process itself.

A Brief Guide to Pursuing a School Evaluation

As can be seen from Sam's story, getting an evaluation through the school can be extremely useful. Even though it didn't result in a diagnosis, it did provide a template for services for Sam. If you're considering pursuing testing through the school, here are the basic facts.

The first thing you'll want to do is to make a referral, or request for testing, to the special education department for your school system. You should call the special education office of your school district with this request and then follow up with a written letter restating your request for the evaluation. It's also a good idea to let your child's teacher know that you've done this. (In fact, it's a really good idea to have a conversation with your child's teacher even before you make the referral for testing.) Once the school gets your request for an evaluation, it should contact you.

State law may require that the school district respond within a certain time frame; the period may vary from state to state. If you don't hear from your school within a week or 2, you should definitely follow up on your request.

Because you may not know what kind of evaluation your child might need, you may want to request a *preevaluation conference*. This is a meeting between you and at least one member of the special education team, usually the chairperson, to talk about your concerns. You will discuss what kind of testing will be helpful, and who will be doing the evaluations at school. Though the specific types of evaluations may vary from child to child, *you should always request that a full intelligence measure be given to get an estimate of your child's potential.*

The intelligence tests that are most frequently administered to school-age children are the Wechsler Intelligence Scale for Children, Fourth Edition (WISC-IV); the Differential Abilities Scale, Second Edition (DAS-II); and the Stanford–Binet Intelligence Scales. You'll also want to make sure that *processing speed is thoroughly evaluated* within the context of the evaluation. More information about these measures and how to interpret the scores is provided in Chapter 3, but a brief listing of the most commonly used tests is provided below. If school personnel do not have the ability to perform such testing, the district can always send you to an outside evaluator at the school's expense.

Before starting any evaluation, the school district must send you advance written notice about the kinds of testing it plans to do with your child, as well as provide notice of the procedural safeguards available to you (for example, your right to reject testing, confidentiality of student records). Be aware that you have the right to consent to some evaluations but not others. As we noted, Sam's parents decided they wanted a private speech and language therapist to complete that portion of the evaluation with Sam, while they had the school district conduct the rest of the evaluation.

Once you agree with what the school proposes to provide in the evaluation of your child, *you must give written consent before the school will begin the evaluation.* Federal law states that the evalua-

COMMONLY USED TESTS
OF PROCESSING SPEED

Nearly any timed test can be considered some type of a measure of processing speed. In the course of a typical comprehensive evaluation (whether it's a school or private evaluation), a number of timed tests will be given/administered. Some of the more common ones include the following:

Wechsler Intelligence Scale for Children, Fourth Edition (**WISC-IV**). The WISC-IV measures processing speed in a number of different ways, including subtests such as **Coding** (a test where the child is asked to quickly copy a code), **Symbol Search** (where the child is asked to quickly determine whether different symbols are the same or different), and **Cancellation** (where the child is asked to cross out all of the animals on a given page). The WISC also provides a **Processing Speed Index**, a composite score that consists of the average of two of the three previously mentioned subtests.

Differential Ability Scales, Second Edition (**DAS-II**). Similar to the WISC, the DAS provides individual measures (or subtests) of processing speed, as well as an overall index. The individual subtests include **Speed of Information Processing** (where, for example, the child is presented with rows of numbers and asked to quickly cross out the biggest number in a row) and **Rapid Naming** (where the child is asked to name as many items in a given category, such as colors or animals) as quickly as he can.

Woodcock–Johnson Test of Achievement, Third Edition (**WJ-III**) *Academic Fluency Subtests.* The WJ-III includes subtests that measure math, reading, and writing fluency. The child is asked to compute numbers, read and answer questions about a passage, or compose sentences, all within a limited time period. These individual measures can be combined into a global measure of academic processing speed or academic fluency. The *Wechsler Individual Achievement Test* (**WIAT-III**) has similar subtests (**Math Fluency** and **Reading Fluency**) that measure how quickly a child is able to perform math and reading skills.

Other popular tests of processing speed include *Trail Making Tests* (where the child connects dots or patterns in a certain order), *Stroop Tests* (where the child rapidly reads words or names colors), and *Grooved Pegboard Tests* (where the child puts pegs in a pegboard as quickly as possible).

tion must be completed within a reasonable period of time after the school receives the parent's consent; the law of your state may specify a particular number of days within which the school must complete all necessary evaluations. The child must be assessed in all areas of suspected weakness or disability; thus, depending on the concerns that brought you to this evaluation, more than one type of evaluation may be needed. Often the school system will provide a multidisciplinary evaluation, which is a comprehensive assessment that usually includes several professionals such as school psychologists, occupational therapists, reading specialists, speech and language therapists, and physical therapists.

A Brief Guide to Pursuing an Independent Evaluation

The trickiest part of pursuing an independent evaluation is finding a competent evaluator. The professionals who are most qualified to evaluate processing speed in children are *child psychologists*. Finding a child psychologist might sound like a simple task, but it's not, for a couple of reasons. It may surprise you, but the need for child psychologists far outweighs the number of available professionals who are trained in this area. This gap is true across the country, and some parts of the country (particularly rural areas)

WHO IS QUALIFIED TO ASSESS PROCESSING SPEED?

Child Clinical Psychologists

- Psychologists have a doctorate degree and have completed at least 4 years of specialized graduate school training (after completing college) and 2 years of full-time supervised clinical experience after graduate school.

- Since this book relates to childhood concerns, you'll want to make sure you find a clinical psychologist who was specifically trained to treat and assess children (as opposed to adults).

- Not all child clinical psychologists have completed specialized training in child testing and assessment, so you'll want to make sure you find someone with this type of training.

Pediatric (or Child) Neuropsychologists

- Clinical psychologists who have completed specialized training in using neuropsychological tests to evaluate intellectual, memory, language, and visual–motor skills (among others) in order to diagnose problems such as learning disabilities, attention problems, and developmental disorders.

- Not all neuropsychologists have specialized training in assessing children, so make sure you find someone who has extensive experience with pediatric populations.

School Psychologists

- School psychologists work in school settings and are generally trained to provide counseling to children as well as to administer tests of intellectual functioning and academic achievement.

Educational Psychologists

- Educational psychologists are psychologists trained in improving curricula, teaching methods, and adminis-tration of academic programs.
- Educational psychologists are rarely trained to admin-ister tests and provide diagnoses, but some are. You'll need to check their credentials to determine whether this is the case.

have an even smaller number of clinicians who are trained to treat and evaluate children. You'll also want to make sure you're seeing a psychologist who has specialized in the *assessment* of childhood psychological disorders as opposed to the *treatment* of childhood disorders.

As you can see in the sidebar above, there are different types of psychologists, any of whom may be trained to administer tests and provide assessments. Clinical psychologists and neu-ropsychologists have doctorate degrees (PhDs), whereas school and educational psychologists may or may not have a doctorate. (Requirements for licensed school psychologists vary by state, with most states requiring at least a master's degree for licensure or certification.) Child psychologists most often work in either hospital or clinical settings.

So, given that there are few clinicians and that they may have different titles, how does a parent find a competent professional? Your first stop could be your child's pediatrician or primary-care physician, as pediatricians usually have a list of referrals they use in these situations. Similarly, professionals at your child's school may have recommendations. This is particularly true if your child attends a private school, because private schools often have a number of professionals with whom they have working relationships. Word of mouth is also a great way to get a recom-mendation. If you know friends, relatives, or neighbors who have had their child tested—and you feel comfortable discussing your child's issues with them—ask them who they used and what the experience was like.

Once you've made the appointment, expect the evaluation to take 3–6 hours, depending on the age of the child and the areas that need to be assessed. Some evaluators complete the evaluation within the course of a single day, whereas others have children come for testing on multiple days. There is no one "right" way to complete an evaluation. Experienced evaluators have good reasons for their procedures (that is, what works for them and/or their clinic). After the evaluation, the psychologist will summarize the results in a comprehensive written report that you should receive. The psychologist will typically meet with you to review the results and, depending on the age of your child, sometimes

"I finally found a child psychologist who seems like the perfect person to evaluate my daughter. Unfortunately, the psychologist said she doesn't have any availability for 4 months! What's the deal with that?" A 4-month wait time for a private evaluation is not uncommon; in fact, we'd say it's the norm as opposed to the exception. In many clinics a 6- to 12-month wait is typical. This is one area in health care where the demand for services far exceeds the supply. However, if you've found someone you really like, it's usually better to spend extra time waiting for him or her as opposed to seeing someone who isn't as well qualified but who has immediate availability. Just because you're waiting for an evaluation doesn't mean you can't do something in the meantime. Talk to your child's teacher to get ideas about what can be done for your child while you're waiting for the evaluation appointment. Ask to be on a cancellation list (and be prepared to take an appointment at a moment's notice). When making the appointment with the professional, ask him or her if there are things, such as reading or math tutoring, that you could do for your child while you're waiting for the appointment.

review the results with your child as well. In the next chapter, we provide information on how to understand the test results, but you shouldn't be afraid to ask questions of the evaluator if there are things you don't understand. Understanding what the results mean is the basis for making sure you can adequately advocate for your child.

Where Do You Go from Here?

Whether or not you've decided on getting an evaluation, you most likely picked up this book because you wanted a better understanding of your child and some ideas on what to do. If your child has had an evaluation, whether through the school or independently, you should have a road map as to where to go from here. If you've pursued an evaluation and *don't* feel like you have any ideas about where to go, ask the evaluator for more information or get a second opinion. Parents are rarely wrong when they think their child needs help. If you've had an evaluation and were told your gut instincts were wrong, chances are you need more information—either as to why your instincts are incorrect or why the results show no cause for concern.

In any case, you are likely wondering what you should—or can—do now that you have identified a specific area of concern. Although Part II of this book discusses how to cope with processing speed deficits in a variety of settings, including home, school, and social settings, before going into more detail we'd like to give you some basic *dos* and *don't*s to help frame your thinking about basic problem areas and general solutions.

Accepting your child's unique learning style, helping her to *accommodate* any learning challenges, and *advocating* for your child's needs are good places to start when thinking about solutions. We call these the *three A's of processing speed*. In some ways, these ideas might be obvious—most parents do these things naturally; good parents are accepting, accommodating, and advocate for their children when needed. When your child has a weakness, particularly one that is as hard to pin down or define, as process-

THE THREE A'S
OF PROCESSING SPEED

1. **Accept:** Get information about your child's learning profile so that you can better understand his unique qualities and *accept* those qualities as being an important—and valuable—part of who he is.
2. **Accommodate:** Find ways to modify your child's environment so her processing speed weaknesses are accommodated. In addition, help her develop compensatory strategies so that she can learn to make accommodations for herself.
3. **Advocate:** Understanding how your child's learning "speed" affects him in various environments allows you to be an important advocate within and outside the school environment, by developing a plan with the school and helping others better understand your child. The ultimate goal is for you to teach your child how to understand and advocate for himself.

ing speed is, these simple terms carry even more importance and can be harder to implement.

It's easy to accept your child's performance when he's the first to hit a home run on the baseball field, but more difficult to accept his behavior when he's taken 30 minutes to do one simple math problem, and he still has 14 problems left to complete on the homework sheet before tomorrow. If a math curriculum isn't challenging enough for a child, it's much easier to advocate for her to be given a more complex curriculum than it is to ask that she have fewer homework problems to complete because it's taking her 3 hours to do a math worksheet that should take 20 minutes. It'd be a whole lot simpler to accommodate your child's slowness in getting ready for school in the morning if you didn't have two other children who needed help and a boss who expected you to get to work on time.

Responses You Wish You Hadn't Used

These responses may be similar to some of the challenges you've faced. In fact, they may cause you to feel so frustrated that you've found yourself doing some things you're ashamed to admit. What are the most common offenses? They include things like the following:

YELLING! SCREAMING! SHOUTING!

It's probably not an exaggeration to say that every parent (even ones who have children with fast processing speed) has resorted to these techniques, and we don't need to tell you that they don't generally work. When we say that they don't "generally" work, we're actually saying that they sometimes *do* work—but they don't work *well*. You might yell, and your child might be motivated to act, but the next time you want him to do something, you might need to scream louder or yell for longer. In addition, yelling and screaming can actually slow processing speed because it can make your child anxious, which is likely to further slow down a child's processing speed. These tactics can also make you feel guilty about your behavior—and the last thing a good parent needs is to feel guiltier!

REFERRING TO YOUR CHILD AS "LAZY"

When a child takes longer to complete tasks than her peers, adults frequently comment that she seems "lazy." In fact, many parents— even when they know their child can't go any faster—still *feel* that their child is lazy. Their child procrastinates, has trouble self-starting, makes careless errors in her work, and attempts to take shortcuts. All of these would appear to fall under the definition of "laziness," but there is usually another reason for the behavior, be it depression, inattention, anxiety, lack of self-confidence, or a slower processing speed. Your child isn't choosing to act in a way that appears lazy. Instead, her behavior is more likely a symptom of an underlying issue that needs to be addressed.

COMPLETING WORK FOR YOUR CHILD

Parents of children with weak processing speed frequently complete work for them. In fact, many parents complete schoolwork for their children—and they don't want to admit it. Of course you know that it's a bad habit to get into, but what can a parent do when the assignment is due tomorrow and there's no way your child can get it done? Hopefully this book will give you some concrete strategies, but, given the fact that you'll probably do this at one time or another, you need to be very aware of *when* you tend to do this (only at the last minute), *what* you're doing (is it only math homework, writing assignments, or everything?), and *how* you're doing it (are you giving support or are you actually doing the whole assignment?). Examining these issues can be very helpful in determining how to help your child.

Perhaps the most important thing to keep in mind is that *accepting, accommodating,* and *advocating* are lifelong processes that parents struggle with—and learn from—as they watch their children grow from infancy to adulthood. If you've got a child who is particularly challenging, you're just more aware of how hard it is to put these simple terms into practice on a daily basis. More than once we've heard the saying "The days are long but the years are short" applied to parenting. This is particularly true if your child seems to take a really long time to get things done. An evening of homework can seem like an eternity, and these day-to-day struggles might make you feel you have little time left to actually enjoy life with your child so that the years seem to be flying past far too quickly.

You're not alone. Most parents feel this way at one time or another. Taking the long view and understanding and accepting that this is part of the parenting process can be helpful to keep in mind. Knowledge is the beginning of acceptance. Without it, there is little ability to know how to accommodate or advocate. The next chapter provides you with more information—and knowledge—so that you can better understand this topic and see it as a normal part of who your child is. He's not lazy, incompetent, or dumb; she is not just acting this way so that the whole family is miserable. Your child is just different—and for him or her, being *different* is *normal*.

three

"So What, Exactly, Is Processing Speed?"

Parents have asked us many questions over the years, such as "Will my child ever learn to read?" or "Why doesn't my child have any friends?" or "Is my child depressed?" Although these are difficult questions to answer, no question is more difficult for us to answer than "What exactly is processing speed and is there any way to fix it?" A few parents are happy enough with our defining processing speed as "how long it takes your child to complete a task within a certain amount of time." Other parents seem satisfied with the idea that processing speed is thought of as an *executive function* skill—a group of skills that allows us to use our intelligence efficiently. But most parents want a more comprehensive explanation to a problem that seems to impact every aspect of their child and family's life.

Our goal in this chapter is to try to give you a more complex answer to the question of "What is processing speed?" by reviewing what we know about how the brain processes information and by what we're learning from our own studies here in our clinic. But first, it might be helpful to know a few facts about why we know so little about this important topic.

WHAT ARE EXECUTIVE FUNCTION SKILLS?

Executive function skills allow us to successfully use our intelligence and problem-solving abilities. These skills include abilities such as goal setting, planning, organizing, prioritizing, remembering information in working memory, monitoring our behavior, and shifting back and forth between different tasks or activities. Processing speed is considered an important executive function skill.

"So is processing speed just another word for executive functions?" No, but here's a good way to think about it. Imagine that executive functioning is the car, and processing speed is the engine. Having a faster engine or a more powerful engine means the car can go faster, so good executive function depends on the quality of the engine. More efficient engines allow the car to function at a higher level of efficiency.

The History of Our Concept of Processing Speed

The idea of processing speed may seem new to you, but it's actually been around for a long time. Some of the earliest studies in psychology investigated processing speed and its relationship to intelligence. In the late 1800s the first studies on processing speed considered individual differences in reaction times. These tests included measures that examined how quickly someone reacted to sounds or noise of some kind, as well as other mental tasks such as how many numbers someone could remember after hearing them only once.

Sir Francis Galton (who also happened to be a cousin of Charles Darwin) was one of the first people to assert that mental processes (such as intelligence) could be measured quantitatively. In 1884, at the International Exhibition in London he presented a series of experiments that the general public could experience firsthand. These experiments measured different types of reaction times as they related to how quickly someone perceived something or reacted motorically to something. During this time period, studying reaction times was widely accepted as a way to measure variabilities in people's mental processes. It was a popular topic among the general public. Some researchers at the time thought that measuring differences in processing speed would revolutionize assessment and psychology as a whole. In fact, some were so bold as to assert that processing speed could predict how successful people could be (although "success" was not specifically defined).

Despite these bold ideas, as psychology advanced into the 1900s, the idea of studying processing speed fell out of favor. Younger researchers began to examine the relationship between reaction times and found virtually no relationship between these types of tests and students' abilities, as measured by their grades in school, and therefore made the assumption that such tests were not valid measures for predicting intelligence. By the 1920s,

IS PROCESSING SPEED JUST ANOTHER TERM FOR REACTION TIME?

The answer to this question is *no*. Reaction time is part of processing speed, but processing speed also includes how quickly a child:

- Integrates new information
- Retrieves information from memory
- Performs certain tasks

It can be visual, verbal, or motoric (or include all three), and it can be content-specific (reading, writing, motor, math), although a child with slow processing speed will often show problems across a number of areas.

the study and clinical assessment of sensory processing speeds as a way to measure intelligence was brought to a standstill by inconclusive research studies such as the ones indicated above.

Psychology then started to move away from these types of basic scientific studies toward more Freudian-type theories about the unconscious and psychoanalysis, as well as examining ideas about how our behavior is controlled by reinforcement and punishment. For decades, processing speed was not regarded as an important topic to study within the field of psychology. This is why processing speed has been an understudied topic compared to topics such as language or memory.

However, the past few decades have brought a resurgence of interest in processing speed from both a research standpoint and a "real-world" standpoint. In terms of the research context, scientists have started to examine the biological systems that control our behaviors and emotions, and mental speed has become an area of interest within this field. For the first time, brain-imaging research can look at how—and *how quickly*—a brain can process information. In addition, more recent theories of intelligence have incorporated speed, in various forms, as a major component in intelligence testing. The Wechsler scales of intelligence include processing speed as a major index, and researchers—and parents—are asking the question "What is the meaning of this factor, and how does it relate to intelligence and functioning?"

At the same time, our world has become more fast-paced. In order to be successful in today's world, you need to be able to process large amounts of information quickly and to be able to shift back and forth between different types of tasks. Processing speed is now something that is being discussed in schools and research labs as an important issue to understand.

The Biology of Processing Speed

No single brain region has been (or is likely ever to be) identified as the problem with processing speed. As it is with most higher brain functions, one's abilities in processing speed involve a complex network of different parts of the brain, all acting in concert. As you can see in the diagram below, the brain is composed of different lobes. The largest part of our brain is called the *cerebral cortex,* and it's the part of our brain that gives us our distinctly human qualities such as the ability to plan ahead, to reason, and to create. The cerebral cortex is divided into two hemispheres, the right and the left. The left hemisphere plays a big role in language functioning, whereas the right hemisphere's specialty is in social perception, creativity, and nonverbal problem solving.

Other parts of the brain are important too, but the cerebral cortex, and particularly the frontal lobes, is worth special attention. The frontal lobes contain the functions underlying most of our thinking and reasoning ability, including memory. They help us make sense of the world around us, prioritize what's important for us to know, and relate appropriately to others. These functions continue to mature well into late adolescence and early adult-

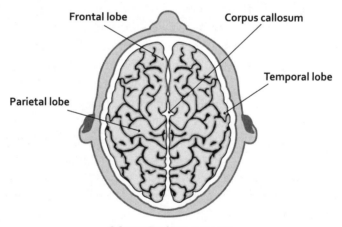

© Gregory Dyer | Dreamstime.com

Parietal lobes: Integrate auditory, visual, and tactile signals; immature until age 16.

Frontal lobes: Important for self-control, judgment, emotional regulation; restructured in teen years.

Corpus callosum: Important for intelligence, consciousness, and self-awareness; reaches full maturity in 20s.

Temporal lobes: Emotional maturity; still developing after age 16.

hood, so the brain your child has now is not the one he'll have when he finishes college.

Differences in speed of processing cannot, at this time, be "mapped" onto different areas of the brain. Instead, it's what we describe as a "global" concept that affects the way the entire brain processes information. Differences in speed of processing may be most related to how well the brain is "wired"—for example, the size of the nerves in the brain, how well the brain metabolizes glucose (the brain's "fuel"), and the integrity of how rapidly and efficiently the brain cells "fire." Each of these components has been shown to affect processing speed, but none alone explains the causes of processing speed.

Overall, though, a number of recent studies of processing speed and the brain seem to converge on the idea that there are some sort of global, biologically driven mechanisms that limit the speed at which information is processed, the most important of those being:

- *Neurotransmitters in the brain,* the biochemical currents in our brain that help us make meaningful connections

- *How well the neurons, or cells, of the brain are covered with myelin*

- *The size of the gaps between the nerves and the nerve receptor sites*

- *How well the neural networks are organized*

- *The efficiency of the frontal lobes in organizing and directing information flow.*

We realize this is a complicated list to digest, so let's discuss each one of these factors in more detail.

NEUROTRANSMITTERS IN THE BRAIN

Neurotransmitters are chemicals in the brain that act like messengers, relaying signals between brain cells (called *neurons*). The brain uses neurotransmitters to tell our hearts to beat, our stom-achs to digest, and our muscles to flex. In addition, neurotransmit-ters control and affect our moods, sleep cycles, weight gain or loss, memory storage and retrieval, and yes, even processing speed.

The brain has at least 100 billion nerve cells, or neurons, and each neuron consists of a body that trails off into a tail (called an *axon*). Axons transmit electrical impulses away from the cell body, and something called *dendrites* transmits electrical impulses toward the cell body (see the diagram of a neuron on the facing page). If this sounds complicated, think of it this way: All brain cells consist of a head and tails. Some tails transmit impulses away from the cell, and others bring impulses toward the cell. These cells are very close to one another, but they're not touching each other, so their electrical impulses can't travel over connected tissue; instead, the impulses flow across the space between the neurons. You might be asking yourself, "If these cells aren't con-nected to one another, how do these impulses get from one cell to another—how do they flow across the space?" They are able to communicate through chemicals called *neurotransmitters*. At least seven different major transmitters are currently known to have an effect on perception, motor activity, sensation, emotion, atten-tion, and cognition.

Each of the neurotransmitters seems to have a different major function, and all of the neurotransmitters are necessary in exact proportions for maximal brain functioning. Having too much or too little may be related to genetic, biological factors or to environmental factors, but regardless of the reason, when levels of certain neurotransmitters are low, concentration can be affected and the speed at which information is processed can be slowed. One particular neurotransmitter that has been linked to processing speed is *acetylcholine*. Acetylcholine is involved in increasing or accelerating our responsiveness to sensory stimuli in the environment and is critical for decision making, sustaining attention, and memory. Research has found that low levels of ace-tylcholine in the brain have been linked to slower reaction times, poor attention, and delayed information processing.

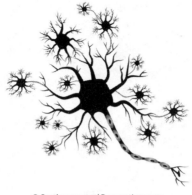

© Svetlanamaster | Dreamstime.com

THE FATTY COVERING OF NEURONS

As the brain matures, the axons of the brain (those "tails" that we referred to on page 46) become coated with a fatty substance called *myelin*. Myelin acts as insulation to improve the efficiency of the signal that is sent between the neurons, much in the same way that electrical tape insulates electrical impulses; see the diagram on page 48. The myelin coating is such a vital part of the neurons in the brain because it allows electrical impulses to flow more quickly and directly from one neuron to another. The amount of myelin that surrounds neurons differs both at varying stages of life and from person to person. Myelin production begins in the womb (as early as 14 weeks after conception) and continues to develop through childhood and into adolescence. One theory for slow processing speed is that the layer of myelin around the brain's neurons may actually be thinner than the average person's. Thus, the less myelin, the slower the message sent—which translates to a slower speed of processing in the brain.

THE SIZE OF SYNAPTIC SPACES

Another biological factor thought to impact processing speed is the size of the space between neurons. This is technically referred

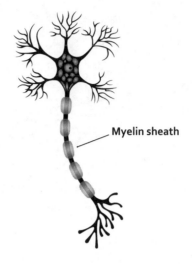

Myelin sheath

© Alila07 | Dreamstime.com

to as the *synaptic cleft,* and it is depicted in the diagram below. The end of one neuron communicates with an adjacent neuron by releasing an electrical current, and neurotransmitters, into the synaptic cleft. These neurons "travel" across the synaptic cleft to the edge of another neuron and "activate" it. The size of the synaptic clefts is important because if the cleft is very large, it will take the neurotransmitters longer to travel across it and activate the adjacent neuron. Some researchers believe that individuals with slower processing speed have larger-than-expected clefts between neurons. Because the neurotransmitters have farther to

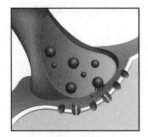

© Tracey Cox | Dreamstime.com

travel from one neuron to another, messages are sent more slowly in the brain.

THE ORGANIZATION OF NEURAL NETWORKS

As you now know, neurons communicate with each other, and when they do, they start to form pathways, or *neural networks*. These pathways are the basis for how the brain works because they control complex activities such as speaking as well as more basic activities such as gripping an object or chewing food. Babies are constantly developing new neural networks. You can almost *see* them making those connections when you watch them repeatedly try to reach for something or imitate a word.

The good news is that we continue to develop new neural pathways throughout our lives. When you first learn something, the pathway or connection is weak, but the more frequently you think of a particular topic, the stronger the pathway becomes. For example, let's say your child is learning to ride a bike. At first she has to pay attention to staying balanced, keeping her eyes on the road, and holding on to the handlebars. The more she practices, though, the less she has to concentrate because the connections formed in the brain for this action have become stronger. Similarly, let's say you're trying to learn Italian for the first time. As you study Italian, the language neurons in your brain that are storing your English language "data" will start to make new connections to other neurons, and these new neural pathways will begin to acquire and store the new language. These new pathways become stronger the more they are used.

On the other hand, let's say there is a "kink" or glitch in one of these somewhat well-established pathways. These glitches can include the types of problems we mentioned earlier (large synaptic clefts or thin layers of myelin), or they can include just poor wiring—that is, the "wiring" of the neural network itself can be faulty. The poor wiring might occur because the task was learned poorly to begin with or because it wasn't practiced enough. Whatever the reason, poor wiring can slow down the processing of information considerably. In terms of a lack of practice, if a certain pathway is activated once, it is easier to activate a second time, third time, and so on. Things do speed up with practice, and some kids need more practice than others. We believe that some kids—those with processing speed deficits—need to *overlearn* a task to perform it efficiently. For these networks to perform efficiently, a child with slow processing may need more practice than the average kid even after it looks like he's mastered the task.

THE EFFICIENCY OF THE FRONTAL LOBES

Parents frequently ask, "What *part* of the brain is most involved in processing speed?" As the last few pages have illustrated, it's not that one part of the brain is weak, but that parts of the system aren't functioning as strongly. Of all the parts of the brain, the frontal lobes are most involved in the function of processing speed, since they are most important for higher-level cognitive functioning. In addition, they perform some very important general functions, such as:

- The ability to persist on tasks even when we're distracted

- The ability to plan goals and determine possible long-term consequences of our actions

- The ability to generate different possible responses to a problem

- The ability to choose and initiate goal-directed behaviors

- The ability to self-monitor our behaviors and know when those behaviors are adequate or not

Implied within this list is the ability to do these things *efficiently* and quickly, and so processing speed is implicitly linked to each one of these tasks. In terms of the biology of processing speed and frontal lobe functioning, studies have indicated that *decreased volume* of the frontal lobes is related to the speed at which someone processes information. Stated simply, a smaller frontal lobe (as defined by gray and white matter in the brain) *may* mean slower processing, although it's not a perfect correlation by any means. Additionally, people who sustain damage to the frontal lobe, such as from a car accident or sports-related injury, often demonstrate a slower performance on tests of processing speed. Thus, if the pathways of the front lobes are damaged, speed of information processing can be affected.

Putting It All Together

By this point in the chapter you hopefully have a better understanding of the possible causes of processing speed weaknesses, while at the same time realizing that there isn't any one area of the brain that can be pinpointed as the cause of these deficits. Many brain structures or areas affect it. Speed of information processing is affected by the neurotransmitters in the brain, by the fat that covers the neurons that can speed transmission of information, by the size of the synaptic spaces (with larger spaces slowing down information processing), by the organization of neural networks, and by the efficiency of the frontal lobes. Of note, a person with slower information processing may also be physically slow, but physical slowness is not the same as slow information processing. It's possible to have intact (in fact, even strong) physical movements but to process information slowly.

You might be wondering, though, what this actually all means for a person in his daily life. How does this difference in processing speed affect a child cognitively, emotionally, academically? Emerging studies are investigating these issues, and although there are no definitive answers, we can give you a sense of what kids with slower processing speed look like in our clinic's research.

Processing Speed in a Clinical Sample

At the LEAP clinic at the Massachusetts General Hospital, we've collected a sample of 600 families, many of whom have family members with processing speed problems. Our sample included children ranging from ages 2 to 20 years of age, with an average age of 10.4 (and a standard deviation of 3.79 years). Although this research by no means provides the final word on this topic, here are some general themes that seem to be emerging:

- *Boys are more affected by processing speed deficits* than girls are. In our sample, 70% of the children who had a significant processing speed deficits were boys. There may be various reasons for this, ranging from the idea that boys may just be slower at the types of fine motor tasks that measure processing speed or the gender biases in teaching. We'll discuss some possibilities around this topic in future chapters.

- *Social difficulties* are common in about a third of the children with processing speed deficits. We'll talk more about this in Chapter 7.

- *Language impairments* were reported in about 40% of the children with processing speed deficits. This may be due in part to the high number of children with reading- and language-based learning disabilities who also have processing speed deficits.

- About a third of the parents reported *delayed motor development* in their children. This is not surprising, given that we measure processing speed using various types of motor measurements.

- The vast majority of the children with processing speed deficits (77%) were currently *receiving services under an Individualized Educational Plan or 504 Accommodation Plan*— which indicates the level of impact that processing speed has on academic functioning.

- *Having a processing speed deficit is not the same as having ADHD.* Only 61% of the kids with ADHD also had processing speed weaknesses as compared to their age-matched peers. Thus, although many kids with ADHD have problems with processing speed, not all of them do, and as you'll see from the table below, kids with many other presenting problems can have processing speed deficits.

These data show us that processing speed problems cut across and affect academic, behavioral, and emotional difficulties. Moreover, problems with processing speed come with a host of other issues that may also need to be addressed. This is a good reason to identify whether processing speed is the cause of the problems; it allows the issues to be addressed when a solution may have eluded you before. And once you've identified the problem, you should feel an increased sense of hopefulness. All of the diagnoses mentioned in the table have great options for treatment.

Part II explores processing speed in your child's everyday life—how it affects family relationships (including the likelihood that it runs in the family), what it can look like in the domains in which your child functions, how you can help your child keep up, and how it "feels" to have slow processing speed.

Percentages of Children with Slow Processing Speed Who Have Other Diagnoses

Diagnosis	Percentage of children with slow processing speed who meet criteria for this diagnosis
ADHD	61
Reading disorder	28
Math disorder	20
Generalized anxiety disorder	20
Autism/autism spectrum disorder	17
Writing disorder	15
Learning disability, not otherwise specified	15
Bipolar disorder	6
Language disorder	6
Depression	6

Helping Your Child Keep Up in Daily Life

four

Processing Speed in the Family

Now that you have a better understanding of the science of processing speed, you hopefully are developing a foundation of knowledge that can help you support your child. But helping your child also involves helping the whole family, because processing speed doesn't just affect an individual—it's also a *family issue*. When one gear in a machine slows down, the whole mechanism can't work at full potential. When one person is always behind in a family, the rest of the family struggles too, and sometimes it might feel like the whole system has shut down.

On top of that, slow processing speed runs in families, so in some families it's not just one "gear" or person slowing down the process. Now this might sound hopeless, but it's not. In fact, the first step in fixing the problem is noticing not just your child's tendencies, but also your own. In this chapter the focus is on you, the parent, as well as other family members. Understanding the rest of the family is a big step in understanding how to make life easier for everyone.

Slow Processing Speed Runs in Families

There's a reason that sayings such as "Like father, like son" and "The apple doesn't fall far from the tree" are popular. Kids do tend to resemble their parents. Shane was a 12-year-old boy who was just like his dad, but interestingly, Shane's family hadn't really noticed this similarity until they received results of Shane's evaluation. Shane's parents sought an evaluation because he regularly failed to complete his homework and he was often unable to complete his exams in the allotted time. Difficulties finishing homework and tests were having a major impact on Shane's grades, and this issue became a major factor when he got to middle school.

In the course of our evaluation with Shane, we noticed something interesting about his father. Shane's father was slow to fill out questionnaires about his son and was late to appointments at our office. When describing his son's difficulties, we had to explain it in several different ways and draw diagrams to help his father understand Shane's weaknesses. Although Shane's father was not the one being evaluated, we couldn't help noticing that his father struggled with the same issues that Shane did. When we shared our observations with Shane's father, he confessed that Shane was "just like me." Although a successful doctor, Shane's father admitted that it took him hours to complete patient notes and that he often fell behind and had to stay late into the night at the hospital. He had struggled throughout medical school, was slow to complete tests, and was often late to classes.

You might be asking yourself, "So how did he become a successful doctor?" Shane's father was bright, and his intelligence helped him cope with his weaknesses, but another reason was that Shane's father married a woman with very fast processing speed. He dated her throughout college and married her before starting medical school. She helped him in many ways—and was helping Shane too—almost *too* much, and she found herself resenting it. The effects of Shane's slow processing speed, combined with living for years with his father's slow processing speed, was making life miserable for all of them.

It's not surprising that Shane would have a parent with a processing speed deficit; studies have shown that genes from a child's parents may account for 50–70% of processing speed ability. Of course, other factors, such as a stimulating home environ-

DRAW A PROCESSING SPEED FAMILY TREE

Slow processing speed tends to run in families. To trace the path of processing speed, we sometimes ask parents to draw a family tree in our offices. We encourage parents to think about family members, both still living and deceased, and identify those with either suspected or known slow processing speed. Here we provide an example from Nicole's family.

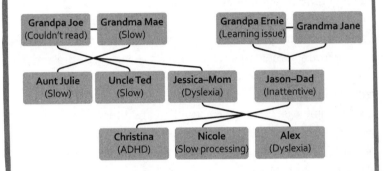

Nicole was a 6-year-old girl who was tested in our offices due to slow progress in first grade. Her parents noted that she was behind in all of the typical skills expected of a first grader, such as learning to read. Teachers commented that it seemed as if the pace of the classroom was too fast for Nicole. We wondered if other family members had similar problems, and we asked Nicole's parents to draw a family tree identifying anyone who seemed similar to their daughter. As Nicole's parents started writing things down, the issues became clearer for them. Like Nicole, there were many family members on both sides of the family who were "slow," "had learning issues," or were identified through testing to have slow processing speed.

ment and the quality of the school environment, are involved in determining a child's processing speed, but genetics are just as important. The link may not be directly from parent to child; there may be aunts, uncles, or grandparents with slow processing speed.

Previous generations would not have labeled this as *slow processing speed*—although they may clearly have described the relative as *slow*. Quite likely they used descriptions such as "Uncle Billy took forever to get anything done" or "Your grandmother would have been late for her own funeral" or "Cousin Bob had so much potential, but he never finished anything."

In our interviews with parents, we often ask them to think about other family members who have a history of slow processing speed. In some cases we even ask the family to draw a "processing speed family tree," which helps us identify links among family members with similar issues.

In some cases, we have actually met children whose parents received some form of testing themselves in the past. Sometimes parents needed testing in school to get into gifted programs, others needed testing to identify a possible learning disability, and others simply had testing as part of their school's standard procedure. If parents have their own test scores available, we encourage them to bring the results when meeting with us because Mom's and Dad's testing profiles may help us better understand their child's profile.

For instance, 10-year-old Eva came to our offices for testing because of problems concentrating in class, trouble getting her homework done, and difficulty picking up on social cues (for example, slow to react to jokes, trouble understanding sarcasm). During the course of Eva's evaluation, Eva's father had found the results from testing he'd had during law school. He remembered that the testing "helped him get extended time on exams" and thought it might aid our understanding of his daughter's problems. Eva's father had been administered an earlier version of the Wechsler Adult Intelligence Scale—Revised (WAIS-R), and Eva was administered the WISC-IV. Following our evaluation, the results were staggeringly similar.

LIKE FATHER, LIKE DAUGHTER

Parents and children may share similar cognitive profiles. Take the case of Eva (age 10) and her father, Stephen (age 44). Stephen had had a full neuropsychological assessment during law school (1996), and Eva had an evaluation in our offices (2013). Results of intelligence testing, including measures of processing speed, are presented below.

The average Composite Score is 100 and scores between 85 and 115 fall within the average range. Stephen's and Eva's results are strikingly similar and show a very significant problem with processing speed. Here are two people who have problem-solving skills in the top 2–3% of the population, yet their processing speed skills fall in the bottom 2–3% of the population. However, in the right field of law, which for him was real estate law, involving a lot of time reviewing details and contracts, Stephen was quite successful—his intellectual skills were valued whereas his processing speed skills weren't as important, or even necessary. Slowly thinking about a problem and a solution was something he did well, and once he found his niche, he was quite successful. He also served as a wonderful role model for Eva.

Measure	Composite score	Percentile
Stephen's WAIS-R, 1996		
Verbal Comprehension	130	98th
Perceptual Organization	129	97th
Freedom from Distractibility	106	66th
Processing Speed	72	3rd
Full Scale IQ	112	79th
Eva's WISC-IV, 2013		
Verbal Comprehension	127	96th
Perceptual Reasoning	129	97th
Working Memory	102	55th
Processing Speed	68	2nd
Full Scale IQ	110	75th

The "Fit" between Family Members

Research has shown that when children are not well matched to their environment, they can show behavior problems and other difficulties as they grow up. Thus, many psychologists have focused on something called "goodness of fit"—that is, how well children's personalities and behavior match—or *fit with*—their family's. Most research has focused on the fit between parent and child, as opposed to siblings or extended family, and research has consistently shown that family stress increases when there is a bad fit, or match, between a child's temperament and his parent's.

Although slow processing speed is only one variable, it is an important one, and it's one that becomes increasingly important over time. Many variables, such as the match between a cranky baby and an easily irritated mom, tend to get better over time (that is, the mother learns to be more flexible and the baby matures and becomes less cranky), but processing speed problems tend to become *more* of an issue over time as the expectations to interact successfully in a fast-paced world increase.

It is critical, therefore, for parents to know their own speed of processing, so they can better understand how they are matched to their children. Processing speed might look a little different in adulthood, but the main premise remains the same: It is the *speed at which someone gets things done*. Look at the checklist of what slow processing speed might look like for parents (on pages 63–64). The more checkmarks you make, the more problems you probably have with processing speed. Also, compare the total score to your child's score on the similar checklist in Chapter 1. Comparing these two scores could provide you with insight into where your own styles "match" and "mismatch." It might also be useful for you to complete these checklists for every member of the family, so feel free to photocopy the checklist or download it from *www.guilford.com/braaten3-forms*. Not only compare the total scores (to see how different family members match up), but also consider a person's pattern of strengths and weaknesses and his or her match with other family members' patterns.

What Is *Your* Processing Speed?

Check off all of the following items that apply to you (or to another family member for whom you are filling out the form).

Visual Processing

- ❑ Don't pay close attention to details
- ❑ Don't proofread what I write (for example, e-mails, notes)
- ❑ Make careless errors
- ❑ Miss the subtle cues of social relationships
- ❑ Find myself staring into space instead of looking at important visual information
- ❑ Omit letters, words, or phrases in my writing or typing

Verbal Processing

- ❑ Find myself tuning out or not listening to others
- ❑ Don't seem to understand directions or multistep instructions
- ❑ Become overwhelmed when someone tells me too much information at one time
- ❑ Need a lot of time to make decisions or answer questions
- ❑ Am hesitant to give an answer, even when I know I am right
- ❑ Provide only short answers to questions
- ❑ Don't participate in group discussions at work
- ❑ Can't seem to remember details or recall facts like other people do
- ❑ Can't keep up with the pace of meetings and presentations
- ❑ Make grammatical errors in my writing
- ❑ Have problems sustaining focused attention during social gatherings
- ❑ Am not "quick" in conversation (for example, think of something to say after it's over)

Motor Speed

- ❑ Am tired, even when I've had a good night's sleep
- ❑ Am seen as lazy or unmotivated by others
- ❑ Move slowly

(cont.)

- ❏ Am reluctant to start tasks or projects (for example, making a family album)
- ❏ Can *do* the task, but not in the time that would be expected to get it done
- ❏ Am slow at the physical aspects of writing

Occupational/Academic Fluency

- ❏ Am, and always have been, a slow reader
- ❏ Did poorly on math drills in school and struggle to remember math facts
- ❏ Have difficulty taking notes in meetings
- ❏ Have trouble expressing my ideas in writing
- ❏ Show inconsistent performance at work (for example, 3 slow days, then 1 fast day)
- ❏ Can't read well aloud
- ❏ Become distracted at work
- ❏ Make punctuation and capitalization errors in my writing
- ❏ Make careless spelling errors in writing, despite being a good speller

General Difficulties

- ❏ Others often say I look confused
- ❏ Others complain I am absentminded
- ❏ Lack persistence in completing any type of task
- ❏ Avoid tasks that require sustained attention or focus
- ❏ Generally seem to be "slow" much of the time
- ❏ Need extra time to complete tasks
- ❏ Forget things easily, such as things told to me earlier that day
- ❏ Frequently ask, "What?"
- ❏ Start out strong but then give up
- ❏ Rush through tasks just to get them done
- ❏ Am hesitant to participate in social situations or conversations

The more symptoms you checked off, the higher the likelihood that you also experience some difficulty in processing speed.

FAST PARENT—SLOW CHILD

One of the most common parent–child "mismatches" we see in our offices is a *fast parent* with a *slow child*. Parents arrive to the office visit with paperwork organized and speaking quickly, while fielding e-mails from work on their iPhones, as their children lag behind, forgetting their backpack in the waiting room, adding long pauses before answering our questions, and seeming unclear about the whole reason they are in our office. For parents with fast processing speed, having a child with slow processing speed can be very frustrating—and for children with slow processing speed, having a fast parent can be equally trying.

Michael was a 13-year-old who arrived with his mother 45 minutes late for his appointment because Michael forgot to come home after school. He and his mother argued about who was to blame for their tardiness. "I was chillin', Mom," he said, "and you need to learn how to chill too!" His mother, a high-powered business executive, was anything but "chill." She managed more than 500 different clients at a time, was early for appointments, and was highly organized. She had completed business school a year early and described herself as running her home "like a well-oiled machine." She could not understand why Michael was so slow and described him as being just like her brother-in-law—Michael's paternal uncle.

We conducted a full neuropsychological evaluation of Michael in our offices, and the results showed that he met criteria for the inattentive type of ADHD (or ADD). As is the case for many children with ADD, Michael showed extremely slow processing speed. His mother was not surprised. However, she was surprised by our explanation of Michael's difficulties; his slow processing was biological in nature—simply the way his brain was wired. His difficulties were not due to motivation, lack of effort, or low intelligence; it just simply took him longer to get things done.

Almost as important as identifying Michael's issue was helping his mother understand the mismatch between her processing speed and Michael's. We highlighted the frustration this was causing for both of them, and they agreed. Next we helped Michael's mother set realistic expectations for her son. We pointed out that yelling and demanding that Michael "move faster" were likely counterproductive. Further, we began to broach the notion that Michael might not grow up to be the high-powered *fast-paced* executive that she was; his cognitive style was just not well matched for that kind of job. In the process, his mother shared with us her fears that Michael would grow up to be "just like his dad," a musician who never was very successful because he could never get things done. She had divorced Michael's father for many reasons, but admitted that one of them was so that Michael wouldn't turn out like his father.

We assured her that slow processing speed is not a recipe for an unsuccessful life. However, not understanding who you are—and being criticized by parents and teachers for things you can't entirely control—can lead to negative consequences. These insights helped modify Michael's mother's expectations, provided insight into why family life had been so stressful, and ultimately helped Michael and his mother understand each other better.

SLOW PARENT—SLOW CHILD

Another possible parent–child combination is a *slow parent* and a *slow child*. This match is fairly common, given the genetic roots of processing speed. Although a slow parent and slow child combination sounds like it could be a good match in which the parent might be more understanding, in reality it can result in two people who are equally frustrated with one another.

Lisa, 11 years old, and her mother, Darlene, exemplified the problems arising from two slow processors. Darlene described Lisa as a "walking disaster" who couldn't finish tests, complete projects, or get up on time. Lisa was in detention at least once every 2 weeks for being tardy to class. Darlene confessed that she had many of the same issues and had just been dismissed from her job as an administrative assistant to a banking executive because she was chronically behind in nearly every aspect of her job. Darlene also revealed that the house was a "disaster," noting that she began a renovation of the kitchen she had never finished.

The wood flooring she and her husband were going to lay was still sitting in boxes in the middle of the living room. Testing revealed that Lisa had slow processing speed, as well as problems with attention and executive functioning (for example, planning ahead, organizing, seeing the "big picture").

In the process of discussing Lisa's test results with her mother, Darlene shared with us that she had lost her job because she had some of the same problems that Lisa had. We talked about how that *could* put Lisa at a disadvantage because it's hard for Darlene to know how to help since they were so much alike— and because Darlene hadn't yet learned the skills that we hoped Lisa would learn. Lisa needed someone in her life to provide structure, routine, and clear expectations, and so did Darlene. Given that we knew it would be difficult for Darlene to help Lisa compensate for her slow processing speed and executive function weaknesses, we recommended that Darlene find an executive functioning tutor for her daughter—someone to help keep Lisa organized, study effectively, and complete tasks on time. The idea here was to *outsource* the help for Lisa's processing speed and thereby relieving pressure on Darlene to compensate for Lisa's weaknesses. We also shared with Darlene that it wasn't too late for her to learn some coping strategies as well, and we provided her with a referral for an executive function "coach" who worked with adults with similar needs as hers.

FLEXIBLE PARENT—SLOW CHILD

The best match for a child with slow processing speed is not a parent who is exceptionally fast or slow but a parent who is *flexible*. Josephine was just that type of parent. She instinctively knew when her son Patrick needed motivation to help him get things started, or when he needed some extra time to settle in, or when he needed her direct help. It's not that Patrick only needed more time or always needed her help to finish a project—it's that he needed different things at different times, and she was able to anticipate those needs.

You might be asking yourself, "Does such a parent even

exist?" And the answer is, "Not every hour of every day." It's impossible for any parent to be flexible all the time, but it is something that we can aspire to, and something that can make a very big difference in the life of a family. Flexibility means not saying, "The last time Patrick had a project, it worked perfectly for me to help him in this way—but *it's not working this time, so he's being difficult.*" Instead, say, "For some reason what worked last time isn't working this time, *so what is different this time that's making it more difficult for him?*" Then use that information to anticipate the kinds of problems that might arise for Patrick the next time. If you have more than one child, you might notice that you're a more flexible parent with one child than another because of the differences in their temperaments and personality styles. We've heard parents say, "I'm a much better parent to my other child because I 'get' who she is. I just can't be flexible with my son, who is not like me."

This type of flexibility might be the easiest for a parent who isn't on one of the extreme ends of the processing speed spectrum but, instead, is somewhere in the middle. Being in the middle can allow parents to be fast during times when being fast is helpful and slow when being slow is helpful. But that doesn't mean that only people in the middle are flexible. Regardless of your style, the fact that you're reading this book means that you're seeking answers and wanting information—and that attitude is the foundation for flexibility. We can't be flexible if we don't know *how* to be flexible, or *why* we need to be flexible, or *when* to be flexible. It's our hope that even if we can't provide a how-to list of answers to the questions of *how, why,* and *when,* knowing more about these issues (by reading this book) will give you the ability to think about these things more flexibly.

Laurie, mother of 14-year-old Tyler, was one of the most flexible parents we've ever seen. Tyler had been seen in our offices several times. He was diagnosed with ADHD when he was 8 years old and at that time exhibited impulsive behaviors, temper tantrums, problems focusing, disorganization, and forgetfulness, as well as slow processing speed. At the time of his initial evaluation, Laurie was not the most flexible parent. In fact, when we initially asked why she and her husband had brought Tyler for an evaluation, she said, "Because I can't deal with him anymore." What set Laurie (and her husband) down the path of a more flexible parenting style was the fact that they sought information from a professional and also *implemented the recommendations* they received from the psychologist. This might seem obvious, but not all parents who seek an evaluation for their child necessarily follow through with the recommendations made. Implementing recommendations means modifying your own habits and learned behavior, and making those changes requires flexibility. So if you've already gotten an evaluation but are finding it difficult to implement the recommendations, figure out why it's difficult for you. If you've gotten an evaluation and things aren't better, it's probably time to change course or evaluate why things aren't working. In either of these cases, flexibility is the key ingredient.

As for Tyler, by the time he reached age 14, many of his problems were much less pronounced, and the successful management of his ADHD and slow processing speed deficits were largely attributable to his mother's flexibility. When needed, she functioned as Tyler's "executive functioning" tutor, keeping his notebooks organized, helping him plan for projects, and assisting with his time management. When he was slow to complete his homework, she offered her assistance in getting him started. At other times, when Tyler acted impulsively and rushed through his work, Laurie helped slow him down, speaking to him in a soft voice and telling him to take breaks in between problems. Laurie was quick, fast to react, and organized when needed. She was also calm, slow-paced, and patient when needed. This flexibility—which she worked hard to cultivate—was critical in helping Tyler overcome his processing and attentional difficulties.

SIBLING FIT

Although parent–child fit is important to consider, so is the fit between the processing speeds of siblings. Again, it is the extreme ends of the processing speed spectrum where we see problems. That is, in a family with a slow child, having a sibling that is exceptionally fast or also exceptionally slow can cause difficulties.

Let's first consider the *fast sibling–slow sibling* scenario. This combination can create frustrations for all involved. The fast sibling may feel annoyed that family life needs to be "slowed down" for the slower sibling. The slow sibling may feel as though he cannot keep up with the family and resent the sibling who can get things done easily and quickly. Arguments and frustrations may erupt because of these processing speed differences.

On the other hand, a *slow sibling* paired with another *slow sibling* may be equally difficult. Having multiple children with slow processing speed may slow a family down exponentially. Parents have to split their time and resources helping two or more children cope with slow speed, which can be exhausting. In families where all children have slow processing speed, siblings cannot help compensate for each other or "pick up the slack." Again, like the best parent–child fit, the best fit for a child with slow processing speed is to have a flexible sibling—a sibling who can be accommodating, regulate her own speed to best match the needs at hand, and help compensate for her sibling's processing weaknesses. However, even the most flexible siblings can feel cheated when they are the ones to always have to compromise, so keep in mind that it's hard for everyone—even the family members who on the surface seem to "have it so easy."

THE FIT OF THE WHOLE FAMILY

Though the examples we're provided in this chapter are based on real families, family systems are generally much more complicated than our examples would indicate, and the combinations of the interactions between processing speed styles and family composition (large family, small family, stepparents, stepsiblings) are endless. A family with a fast mother, slow father, fast son, and slow daughter will function much differently than a family with a slow single mother, two slow children, and one fast child.

The Jackson family had a mix of processing speeds. Kelly (Mom) was fast, Jeff (Dad) was slow, Jonathan (son, age 14) was fast, and Leila (daughter, age 10) was slow. It sounds complicated, but the Jackson family was aware of their individual "speeds" and were just naturally good at developing ways of coping with these differences. The Jacksons are what we would call a "flexible family"; they were able to pair off and work with one another in ways that actually supported each other! For instance, it would take Jeff hours to organize family photos on their laptop computer, and Kelly, who was very fast at these kinds of tasks, would get frustrated that it took him so long. She knew it was best not to get involved in these types of projects with her husband because it often led to conflict. So, instead of Kelly working with Jeff on the photo project, Jonathan (who was also fast) would offer to help. Jonathan, who had a very fast processing speed like Kelly, was able to scan visual information very quickly and make fast decisions about which photos should go in which computer folder. And Jonathan actually enjoyed helping his father. It gave him a sense of accomplishment and allowed him and his father to spend some quality time together.

While Jonathan and his father worked on these kinds of projects, Kelly would help Leila with her homework. Although Kelly was fast, she was also the flexible kind of parent (though not always a flexible wife) we mentioned earlier. She was able to slow down her own pace to match that of Leila's ability to complete her homework. Then she would slowly help to move Leila along, redirecting her, pointing out careless mistakes, and giving her lots of encouragement along the way. So, though the Jackson family had a complicated mix of processing speeds, which was often very frustrating, they found ways to cope and support one another.

The Wilson family also had a mix of processing speeds. Leanne Wilson was a single mother, whom her children had nicknamed "the turtle." She was very slow—slow to make dinner, always arriving late to appointments, and very poor at estimating how long something (like a shopping trip) would take. She had two sons, Lawrence (age 12) and David (age 10), who picked up information quickly, didn't have trouble getting through their homework, and loved games where speed was a key component (for example, buzzing in quickly to answer a question). Leanne's daughter, Olivia (age 7), however, was a slow processor like her mother. She needed instructions repeated several times and was slow to answer when asked questions by her mother or teacher.

These different processing speeds made family life stressful at times, and Lawrence and David became easily annoyed during family outings. For instance, they would be ready to run ahead at the science museum, exploring and quickly moving from exhibit to exhibit, while their mother and sister would lag behind, still searching the bag for the water bottle they misplaced. These differences sometimes created a divide in the family. Leanne and Olivia spent more time together because they were more alike and shared common interests, and Lawrence and David were "glued" together almost like twins. They did everything together—videogames, board games, outdoor activities. In the end, Leanne sought consultation from us because she worried about the "disconnects" in the family. Our goal was to help Leanne and her children understand the differences among family members in processing speed (and otherwise) and to come up with strategies to cope with these differences.

How Can the Family Rally Around a Child with Slow Processing Speed?

There are many ways you can rally around your child's slow processing speed. Making use of home supports, school supports, and social supports are all ways to cope, and we'll explore each one of these areas in the next chapters of this book. First, though, we'd like to give you some general ideas to keep in mind. Research in the field of family functioning has identified several steps successful families take to cope with stressful situations. These steps would definitely be helpful for a family coping with the stress of slow processing speed.

ACKNOWLEDGE THE PROBLEM

As is the case for many problems, the first step is acknowledging there is a problem. You're reading this book, so you already suspect a problem, or perhaps even have documented that there is one, and are in the process of accepting what this means for you and your child. If you're having trouble accepting this, there are some things to keep in mind.

First, *not* accepting the problem can lead to years of frustration. For some parents, accepting the problem means accepting that their child is "slower than average on some things," and for some parents this means incorrectly assuming their child is "not smart." By this point we hope we've shown you that these terms are not synonymous.

Second, sometimes parents have difficulty with accepting the situation because they feel that if they do so, they also have to admit that they've *caused* the situation—that they didn't expose their child to a stimulating enough environment, didn't do enough flash cards, or let him watch too much TV. Do know this: *Nothing you've done or haven't done could cause your child to have slow processing speed.*

Finally, sometimes parents have difficulty with acceptance because it's easier for them to think that their child is just "lazy" rather than that she has a chronic issue that will require great flexibility for a large part of her development. Unfortunately, if your child could move faster, she would. No one likes being a step behind, and nearly all children would choose to be faster if they could.

MINIMIZE OTHER FAMILY STRESSORS

It is much more difficult for a family to cope with a child's slow processing speed if there are other significant stressors. Research has clearly demonstrated that coping mechanisms become less effective as the level of stress increases. Thus, it is critical that you identify other forms of stress and attempt to minimize them. Sometimes the most helpful strategy for a child with slow processing speed is minimizing the sources of stress that don't directly involve him. For instance, if you and your husband are going through financial stress, make sure to handle that stress without involving your child in the details of your finances.

EDUCATE, EDUCATE, EDUCATE

Knowledge is power. The more you know, the better your ability to understand and cope with the issues that arise in day-to-day life. You might find yourself less anxious because you do not fear some "thing" that you can't define, but instead have a problem that you feel empowered to cope. You might also find yourself less frustrated and impatient because you'll understand that your child isn't doing this *to* you but instead is only doing the best she can. Taking constructive steps such as reading books like this, consulting with a child psychologist, speaking with teachers, attending local conferences, and talking to other parents are all very good ways of becoming a more educated—and empowered—parent.

So now that we've provided you with information on how to generally cope with the stressors that a child with slow processing speed presents to you and other family members, you might be thinking, "OK, this makes sense, but what can I actually *do* to help?" Being a flexible parent who understands the unique match between family members is a start, but it's not enough. You need some practical and specific techniques too, which we'll explore in the next three chapters of our book.

Processing Speed at Home

If you have a child with slow processing speed, you may find that life at home is stressful and that you often feel overwhelmed and exasperated. In fact, Cheryl's mother, Stephanie, used those exact words to describe her life. We evaluated 11-year-old Cheryl because her teacher thought she had "processing difficulties," and "it never seemed as if she was paying attention to what she was asked to do at school." After school, it would take Cheryl hours to get started on her homework, despite reminders and constant nagging from her mother—and, as Stephanie said, "Forget about asking her to do any chores. We expect her to clean her room and empty the dishwasher, but those things never get done. If she can't finish—or even start—her homework, I can't expect her to help out at home."

Stephanie wondered how it could take Cheryl 30 minutes to simply pick up the laundry off her floor. Cheryl would finally start her homework assignments after dinner, and, as usual, she would have several hours of work—too much to complete before bedtime. Cheryl wouldn't know where to start, and her mother would have to intervene, helping Cheryl take each homework task one at a time. It would take Cheryl an hour to get through a single sheet of math problems, even though the math concepts had just been reviewed at school that day. By the end of the night, both Cheryl and her mother were exhausted and frustrated. School nights were miserable, and Stephanie was desperate for help.

Family life in the 21st century is busy. Parents are juggling a thousand things at once: helping everyone get ready in the morning, making breakfast, coordinating drop-off and pickup schedules, packing backpacks, signing permission forms, checking e-mail, organizing afterschool playdates, making it to dance practice, driving across town to soccer, helping with homework, preparing dinner—the list is endless. Having a child who has processing speed deficits can slow *everything* and *everyone* down. Simple everyday tasks can take twice as long, families run late to commitments, parental frustration escalates into yelling and family conflict, and a child with slow processing speed is left feeling both responsible and frustrated.

Our research has indicated that processing speed is a very big issue in the home. In general, we've found that the slower the processing speed, the more problems are reported with chore completion and daily life. When children with slow processing speed talk about family relationships, they tend to report more negative relationships with their parents at statistically higher levels than their peers. In addition, as seen in the table below, our research shows that the majority of children with slow processing speed have problems at home with a number of different

Percentage of Children with Slow Processing Speed Who Have Trouble with Necessary Functions at Home

Problem area	Percentage who were reported to exhibit significant problems
Staying organized/planning	81
Self-monitoring	76
Getting started on tasks	72
Keeping track of belongings	66
Inhibiting impulses	65
Shifting/transitioning	63

functions, including getting started on tasks, staying organized, and keeping track of themselves and their belongings.

The functions in the table are pretty serious issues, involved in a million home-related tasks, including these:

- Doesn't stay seated during mealtimes.

- Has trouble with changes in routine at home, such as trying new foods.

- Has trouble starting and finishing homework, big projects, and chores.

- Has trouble getting used to new situations, ranging from a new pair of sneakers to a family vacation.

- Acts like a "couch potato."

- Forgets to bring materials home to complete homework.

- Has great ideas for how to be helpful around the house, but lacks the follow-through to enact any of those ideas.

- Underestimates time needed to complete tasks, such as getting ready for school in the morning, getting ready for bed at night, and completing chores.

- Doesn't plan ahead for desired goals, such as saving money for a certain videogame or other big purchase.

- Leaves room a mess and then can't find things.

- Leaves messes that others have to clean up.

- Has trouble recognizing when his behavior annoys others, such as siblings or other relatives.

So, what is a parent to do? Let's revisit the three A's of processing speed introduced in Chapter 2: accept, accommodate, and advocate. In our practice as psychologists, these are our guiding principles for helping families overcome the unique struggles of having a child with slow processing speed.

Accept and Understand How Slow Processing Speed Impacts Life at Home

The first step in finding a solution for a problem is to accept and understand it. Having a child with slow processing speed has significant effects on life at home, and the more quickly you recognize these effects, the more quickly you can address them. Many of the day-to-day effects of your child's slow processing speed may already be obvious to you—although many may not. In our offices, one of the biggest complaints about slow processing speed relates to *homework* time. We admit it: Homework is a pain for all parents. But for parents of children with slow processing speed, homework time can be downright miserable.

HOMEWORK CONFUSION

First, children with slow processing speed often find themselves lost in class; a lesson from the teacher might be presented too quickly or contain too many steps. As a result, when a child arrives home, he can't remember what that homework was about, when it is due, or how the homework is related to the "big picture" (that is, what the whole point of the lesson was in the first place). Because children with slow processing speed have trouble taking in information and retrieving information that they already know, it is common for them to miss the big picture. They're spending so much time trying to process the details that the larger ideas can elude them. This is true even for very bright children who have strong problem-solving skills. Parents may find themselves wondering what is the purpose of the assignment, and may even blame the teacher for giving their child an assignment that seems to have no reasonable goal. But the problem may reside in the fact that their child missed the most important piece of information because he was trying too hard to quickly remember all of the little details.

SLOW STARTING

Second, children with slow processing speed are simply slow to get started on homework tasks. Kyle was an eighth grader with slow processing speed and ADHD, and his parents were extremely frustrated with his "lack of motivation." They saw Kyle as a "lazy" young man, who had problems "self-starting." It would take him over 30 minutes just to get ready to begin his homework. He would slowly get his notebook out of his bag, then realize he was missing one of his textbooks at school. He would then spend time sharpening pencils, texting his friend to ask which pages he was supposed to read, and preparing a snack to eat. Once Kyle actually started his homework, it would take him nearly three times as long as other students to complete the work.

TROUBLE FINISHING

Which brings us to our third point: Children with slow processing speed have marked trouble completing homework, and they (and their parents) are often up until late hours of the night completing homework and preparing for tests.

Although problems with homework completion may be the issue we hear about most frequently in our offices, children with slow processing speed have many other struggles at home. Parents are often frustrated by how long it takes their child to complete simple, day-to-day tasks, such as dressing for the day, getting to the bus on time, and making it to the table when dinner is ready. Jessica, a 7-year-old girl with slow processing speed, had a lot of trouble getting ready for school in the morning. She had difficulty getting out of bed; her parents would wake her and then need to ask her three or four times to get out of bed and get moving. Jessica would slowly make her way to the bathroom, where she would take two or three times longer to brush her teeth than her sister did. She took a long time to get dressed, eat breakfast, and complete her one chore of feeding the dog in the morning.

Like many children with slow processing speed, Jessica

HOW LONG SHOULD IT TAKE TO DO HOMEWORK?

The simple answer to this question is, "It depends," because the completion time for homework is determined by a number of factors, such as grade and type of school (for example, public, private, Montessori). The general standards are this: Younger grades should have a minimal amount of homework (such as no more than 20 minutes a day in first grade), but this will likely build over time. By high school, your child may be spending a couple or more hours per evening on homework. Again, this may depend on how "competitive" the school is and the expectations regarding where students will matriculate.

Schools and individual teachers typically have a target amount of time they expect children to spend on homework. Find out what your school's policy is. If your child is spending much more time on homework than the school is expecting, talk to the teacher about having your child work for an amount of *time* as opposed to doing an amount of *completed work*. You can negotiate this modification informally with your child's teacher, or if that doesn't work or isn't appropriate, formalize it in an IEP or 504 plan.

Knowing that your child will spend only a certain amount of time on homework can sometimes actually speed up her process. For instance, if a child has math homework that is supposed to take the average student 30 minutes to complete but will take her 2 hours, she may be very reluctant to start because she knows there's no way it's ever going to get done. (Most kids can't verbalize this reaction, but they know they are feeling it.) However, if the expectation is that she's only supposed to be spending 30 minutes a day on math, she may very well be more eager to actually start it, and while working on it, she may be more eager to keep going, knowing that there is a clear limit to what she is expected to do.

also had trouble making up her mind and quickly making decisions. For instance, when offered the choice among three different types of cereal, Jessica often stared blankly, seemingly lost in her thoughts. Jessica's parents were frustrated by the fact that they always had to repeat themselves and sometimes wondered whether Jessica was even listening in the first place. It surprised them that Jessica was slow to remember family friends she had already met. Her parents recounted one instance when her mother was chatting with a new neighbor, who had been over to the house and met Jessica several times before. After Jessica's mother and neighbor finished the conversation, Jessica asked, "Who was that, Mom?" Remembering information about family matters, such as rapidly recalling the name of a relative, an upcoming family trip, or quickly recalling meeting someone may prove very difficult for children with slow processing speed.

In addition to taking longer to complete tasks and assignments, kids with processing speed weaknesses have great difficulty *estimating* how long it will take them to complete tasks and activities. That is, when you ask a child with slow processing speed how long it will take to finish her social studies homework, she will likely respond with a drastic underestimate (for example, estimating it will take 30 minutes when it will actually take her 2 hours to complete). Something thought to take an hour turns into 4 hours, and families are left constantly modifying plans and feeling embarrassed, frequently arriving late to events and outings because of poor planning and inaccurate time estimation.

This was the case for 16-year-old Jesse, who was always running behind. When he got home from school, his mother would ask, "How much homework do you have?" Jesse would typically underestimate the time needed to complete his work. "About 45 minutes," Jesse would respond when, in fact, he had over 2 hours of homework—which would take 3 hours for Jesse, given his slow work pace. Consequently, his mother was constantly rearranging plans and canceling appointments. Jesse's poor time estimation, in combination with his slow work speed, was causing great family disruption and frustration.

Jesse's mom called us the week Jesse left for college to let us know that he had made it through high school and was looking forward to college, although she also said that he had yet to send out the thank-you notes for the high school graduation gifts he had received almost 3 months ago. She had been nagging him all summer, and when finally there was only 1 week remaining before his departure for college, he assured her they'd be done before he left, saying, "Mom, don't worry. It'll take me only about 10 minutes to do those. I've got plenty of time." Needless to say, Jesse went to college with 39 thank-you notes left to write.

Accommodate Your Child's Processing Speed Deficits at Home: Strategies and Suggestions

Recognizing the ways processing speed impacts day-to-day life at home is a critical first step in helping your child overcome these weaknesses. As we've mentioned in previous chapters, there is no miracle cure to improve a child's processing speed at home. However, there are several strategies and accommodations parents can use to help their child move more quickly at home, be more efficient, and reduce a family's overall frustration level. As you can see, we have arrived at the second *A* in our three A's of processing speed: *accommodate*.

KEEP THINGS AT THE SAME TIME, SAME DAY, SAME PLACE!

One big problem for children with slow processing speed is that life at home is often not structured or predictable enough, especially in comparison to school. At school, there is a schedule: The plan for the day is often clear, children sit in the same desk and interact with the same people, a teacher closely monitors and attends to students, and each day is similar to the next.

Life outside of school is often much less routine and supervised. The world brings new challenges every day, whether it be making a quick decision about what to order at a restaurant or adapting to a change in plans (for example, going to the movies

JESSE'S POINT OF VIEW

We were curious as to why Jesse thought he couldn't get his thank-you notes done before going to school, so we contacted him to have him explain it from his point of view. His explanation was as follows:

> "Well if I had just sat down and did them, I don't think it would have taken me very long. It would have been better if my mom hadn't said 'Take your time and just do a couple a day over the entire summer.' I think it would have been better if she'd just said, 'Get these done right now!' so that I knew it was something that had a real time limit and that the limit was *now*. Time management is hard, especially when you don't really want to do it, and even though my mom said that I couldn't get it done in 10 minutes, I really do think I probably could have if I hadn't had any distractions. But one day leads to another, and all of a sudden I was in college."

Although Jesse's explanation wasn't completely helpful, it does point out a couple of things. First, even though he didn't get the notes done, he still believed it would have taken him only 10 minutes to write 39 thank-you notes. Second, he did realize that time management is difficult for him, but just noticing that something is difficult doesn't necessarily lead to immediate change—although it's a great place to start. Third, Jesse did give a clue as to what would have been more helpful: his mom needed to be more directive, in this case. She gave him the impression that he had all summer (and he did), but had she said, "Do these today because these people spent money on you and deserve and want to hear how much you appreciate them—and they are expecting notes *now*," Jesse may have gotten the notes done—and, in the process, found that it would have taken him longer than 10 minutes.

> ## PRACTICAL STRATEGIES FOR ACCOMMODATING SLOW PROCESSING SPEED AT HOME
>
> - *Keep things at the same time, same day, same place.*
>   - Establish a clear routine and schedule to increase speed at home.
> - *Change the way you talk at home.*
>   - Modify the rate, tone, and complexity of the way you talk to your children.
> - *Watch the clock.*
>   - Increase your child's awareness of time and assist in time management.
> - *Remember that actions (and visuals) speak louder than words.*
>   - Use both verbal and visual channels to help your child process information faster.

versus the beach, sleeping over at Aunt Wendy's versus Grandma's house). Thus, in our offices, one of the key pieces of guidance we offer parents is to keep the home environment as structured and predictable as possible. Life at home needs to have more of a routine.

Think about it: Practice makes people quicker at completing tasks because the tasks become familiar, predictable, and routinized. Thus we encourage parents to add structure to life at home; keep things methodical so a child with slow processing speed has a chance to "practice" the routine of the day and eventually speed up. Homework should happen in the same place at the same time every night. Hands need to be washed every night before dinner, and everyone should sit in his or her usual spot. Dog food stays in the same closet, and the dog needs to be fed first thing every morning—even on weekends.

Take the case of 10-year-old Tim, who was referred to us by

his parents because they were worried as to why he had difficulty understanding instructions and efficiently completing tasks. Tim and his divorced parents lived a busy life, with both working unpredictable hours. Each day the schedule was different; sometimes Mom would drop Tim off at school, Dad would pick him up from school, and then Dad and Tim would play videogames together until dinner. Then Tim would return to his mother's house and be expected to quickly complete his homework before bed. On other days, the schedule was unpredictably different. His mother would pick him up, and Tim would need to complete his homework early so he could be dropped off at his father's before dinner.

Tim's parents noted how slow-moving he was and how he almost never completed tasks fast enough to get from one place to another. This left Tim and his parents frustrated, and they wondered if the problems were due to their recent divorce. After a formal assessment, Tim's processing speed was found to be much lower than what would be expected for his age. Furthermore, during testing, he had trouble shifting quickly from one activity to another and showed trouble sequencing information. For instance, he had difficulty on tasks of working memory when he was asked to solve a multistep math problem in his head, without the use of paper and pencil. It also took him a long time to move from one test activity to another without needing a break or time to comprehend the instructions of a new task.

We recommended that Tim's parents try to establish a clear weekly schedule and consistency across home environments. We stressed that this structure and predictability would be critical to Tim's success. His parents rose to the challenge, each week creating a calendar for Tim explaining pickup and drop-off schedules. Additionally, Tim and his parents decided on a "homework time" from 3:30 to 4:30 every afternoon, regardless of whether he was at his mother's or father's house. Tim's parents also came up with a structured after-dinner plan: 20 minutes of chore completion (for example, one simple chore per night), an hour of television or videogames, and 30 minutes of reading at bedtime. Tim's parents noticed a big change in his frustration and disobedience. As the weeks went by, he became faster in day-to-day life, rarely getting to school late in the morning, usually starting and finishing homework on time, and transitioning smoothly from one parent's house to another without daily tantrums.

CHANGE THE WAY YOU TALK AT HOME

In our offices, we usually ask parents of children with slow processing speed to stop and think about how they talk to their child at home. Parents are often puzzled by this question. "What do you mean, 'How do I talk to my child?'" they ask. What we want to find out about is (1) the *rate* of a parent's speech, (2) the *complexity* of the language the parent uses, and (3) the *tone* of voice.

For a child with slow processing speed, a quick-talking parent can create great frustration, so the *rate* of speech can be very important. We have met parents who are "circular talkers"; they barely take a breath between sentences to the point where they seem to be talking in circles. Sometimes parents don't even realize how fast they speak until we (gently) help to point it out. Therefore, a very common first step for many parents is to simply slow down the speed of their speech; take more breaths in between thoughts and be more aware of the overall rate of speech.

Parents also need to pace their questions in relation to their child's ability to answer them. For instance, consider the following real conversation between Erica and Allen, Erica's 18-year-old son.

> Erica: So, do you have everything packed for your camping trip this weekend with Matt?
>
> *Three seconds after asking the question, and before Allen has a chance to consider the question and answer it . . .*
>
> Erica: Now where is Matt going to college?
>
> *Three more seconds pass, and Allen still hasn't answered the first question . . .*

ERICA: Well, I'm going to go through your backpack to make sure you've got everything you need.

And off she goes to pack and repack, before Allen even had a chance to consider whether he had everything he needed.

We also often challenge parents to think about the *complexity* of the language they use with their child. Parents are used to asking several questions at once, presenting many directions at a time, giving vague commands, and going off on tangents while they are talking to their children. We all do it. This kind of language doesn't usually pose problems for most children, but children with slow processing speed have trouble with complex language, such as following multistep instructions or following a parent's tangential line of thinking. To make life at home run more smoothly, parents often need to revisit how they give instructions and present ideas to their children.

For example, Kyla's mother was concerned that her daughter's problems following directions were due to defiant behavior. Kyla was diagnosed with "attention and information processing problems" at age 5 years, but now she was 8 years old and her behavior seemed much more troubling. In addition to seeming to "miss" information, Kyla seemed to never do what she was asked to do.

A formal evaluation of Kyla's profile indeed indicated a diagnosis of ADHD and co-occurring problem of slow processing speed. In fact, Kyla's processing speed was at the third percentile—meaning that 97% of other 8-year-old children processed information faster than Kyla. Given her combination of attention difficulties and slow speed of information processing, we wanted to help Kyla's mother find ways to accommodate these weaknesses. As one suggestion, we recommended that Kyla's mother break tasks into smaller components at home, with clear and explicit instructions for each step. Rather than her mother commanding, "Get ready for dance class," and then quickly getting annoyed because Kyla failed to comply, her mother took a new approach. She first asked Kyla to put her dance shoes in her bag.

Next, she asked her to put her tights into her bag. Once complete, she asked Kyla to get an apple from the kitchen pantry. Next, Kyla was asked to put on her jacket and shoes. Finally, her mother instructed Kyla to get in the car. For example, the conversation would go something like this:

MOM: Kyla, it's time to get ready for dance class. Go get your dance shoes and bring them to me. They're in your closet.

Once Kyla found her dance shoes . . .

MOM: Thanks for getting those. Here's your backpack. Go ahead and put them in right here.

Followed by . . .

MOM: Go get your tights. They're hanging up next to the dryer in the laundry room.

Mom is monitoring that Kyla makes it to the laundry room without becoming distracted by things on the way (and redirecting her if she is), followed by . . .

MOM: Great! Now let's get a snack. I'll show you where the apples are in the refrigerator so you can get one to take with you.

After Kyla gets her snack and puts it in the backpack . . .

MOM: It looks like we're all ready for dance class. Now let's put on your coat and boots.

And finally . . .

MOM: Wow! You got ready all by yourself. Let's get in the car.

Breaking the multistep and vague task of getting ready for dance class into individual steps improved Kyla's speed in getting ready and greatly reduced everyone's frustration at home. Does this seem like a lot of work? Probably, but it's a lot less work and frustration than yelling and not getting to class on time.

Like Kyla's mother, parents of children with slow processing speed often find themselves frustrated. So a common strategy that parents fall back on is to yell at their child with hopes of getting the child to move faster and without realizing that the *tone* or the way they convey the information to their child is also important. When parents of children with slow processing speed sound stressed or communicate with a lot of emotion, children often become anxious—which slows them down even further. Therefore, it is important to stay calm and take a few deep breaths when your child is moving slowly or not following instructions. An impassioned and intense tone will only make matters worse by slowing down your child and making you feel guilty.

WATCH THE CLOCK!

Most people find things like clocks, calendars, appointment reminders, and watches helpful. It might surprise you to know that many children with slow processing speed do not find these things helpful and may, in fact, absolutely *hate* the thought of wearing a watch or using a calendar. They don't really understand the concept of time as it applies to how long it will take them to get something done. You'd think that would mean that they'd gravitate toward clocks and timing devices, but it's been our clinical experience that they don't. The clock is sometimes seen as "the enemy"—that is, the means by which they are judged inadequate or to have failed. Thus parents may find themselves in the difficult position of teaching their children how to learn to "watch the clock" even though their child feels that calendars and clocks are "stupid."

As we've said before, the concept of time can be a difficult one for children with slow processing speed to grasp. They will get "lost" in an activity and have no idea how much time has passed. Ian was a bright and diligent student, beginning his homework as soon as he returned home from school. However, as he worked, Ian often became engrossed in the details of his homework—for example, looking up words he didn't know in the dictionary, searching the Internet for additional information

HOW TO CHANGE THE WAY YOU TALK AT HOME

You scream, "I've told you a thousand times today to clean up your room! We have a ton of stuff to do today—we need to be at Grandpa's in about an hour, and you still haven't done a thing I have asked you to do! I give up!"

Note the *rate, complexity*, and *tone* of what has been said and rethink the presentation. Slow down, make the command less vague, and take out the emotion. Try this:

- **Step 1:** *"Julie, we have to leave to go to Grandpa's house in 30 minutes and I really want your room cleaned before we go. Let me help you get started."*

Take a look around the room and decide what's most important to be done and start with that. If dirty clothes on the floor are a "no-no" in your house, start by saying:

- **Step 2:** *"Pick up your pajamas and put them in the hamper."*

Once completed, present Step 3:

- **Step 3:** *"Now let's make the bed."*

You might need to help your child with this task. In fact, it's a good idea to monitor when your child needs help.

- **Step 4:** *"This is looking good, but let's put these toys in the bin before we go so that the dog doesn't chew on them while we're at Grandpa's."*

Once completed, provide a reward (for example, praise, extra computer time).

about topics, and generally showing a slow work pace. He often hadn't realized that hours and hours had passed, and he typically was nowhere near finished with his homework by bedtime.

Ian needed to learn how to pace himself and watch the clock. He also needed to gain an awareness of how much time he was spending on different tasks. We encouraged his mother to help Ian keep track of the time during homework with reminders about the current time and how much time had elapsed. She checked in with him every 15 minutes, wrote down what he was doing at that time, and helped determine whether what he was doing was actually something he *should* be doing. Eventually, Ian started checking in on himself (without his mother's help), but before he could learn the value of doing that, he needed to be shown how it could be helpful.

The other key here is helping your child set appropriate and reasonable time limits for getting homework or chores done. If the expectation is that your child will complete 2 hours of homework per night, help your child stick to this—even if he can't get all the work done in that time. Your child should not be penalized for a slower work tempo. A reduced homework load is something that your child's school may agree to do, particularly in the early grades. You may need to work with teachers to figure out how much homework is appropriate (more to come on this in Chapter 6). The same goes for completing chores around the house. Instead of deciding on a number of tasks to complete around the house, decide on how much time per week you think is reasonable for chores. If you expect your child to complete chores for an hour a week, stick with this time limit. Come up with a few tasks that would be reasonable to complete within the hour, and don't make your child work longer simply because it takes him longer.

As we have said before, time estimation is very tough for children with slow processing speed. When asked how long it will take to complete a task—be it completing math homework, vacuuming the basement, or running to the corner store to pick up a loaf of bread—children and adolescents with slow processing speed will grossly underestimate how long it will take, sometimes erroneously basing their estimates on the average or optimistically thinking that "this time" they will be faster than average. Rarely do they factor in the extra time it will take them to do the task.

Furthermore, we often find kids with slow processing speed have an overly optimistic view of their ability and will think that this time because they are going to "really try hard," they'll be faster than the typical person. They've been told so often, "If you just try harder, you'll get it done faster," that they optimistically think that since they're planning on trying hard this time, it'll be different.

Kendall was a 16-year-old who had great difficulty with time estimation. She ran late to everything—school, field hockey practice, meeting friends at the mall, you name it. We encouraged Kendall and her parents to help make her a TTL, a *timing of tasks list*. First, we had her write down tasks or activities that recur in the week and then, with the help of her parents, record how much time each activity took on a given day (for example, getting ready for school in the morning = 47 minutes, walking from home to school = 15 minutes). Kendall and her family returned to our offices with this TTL, and we were able to create a more realistic daily schedule for Kendall. In many cases, Kendall had not realized how long certain tasks took her. For instance, she had initially told us it took her "less than half an hour" to get ready for school in the morning—though, when she and her parents timed this, it took her over 45 minutes.

ACTIONS (AND VISUALS) SPEAK LOUDER THAN WORDS

Parents of children with slow processing speed frequently feel like their child isn't listening to them. For children with slow processing speed, it can take much longer to "process" what you have said to them, making their reaction time slow or making it appear as though they have not heard what you have said. As mentioned in Chapter 1, children with slow processing speed become overwhelmed with too much verbal information, need more time to answer questions, have trouble keeping up with the flow of conversation, and often appear as though they are not listening. One strategy to improve processing speed is to present information using more than one channel—that is, both the verbal *and* visual channels.

Most teachers of children with attention, learning, or executive functioning difficulties have found it very helpful to teach using more than one sensory channel, such as a combination of verbal and visual learning. Parents can also use this method at home for children with slow processing speed, but it will take a bit of work. Perhaps the most helpful visual aid parents can employ at home is a calendar. This home-based calendar shows the schedule of the day for family members and helps to promote speed at home. It allows a child with slow processing speed to develop routines, which can result in a quicker pace to the day because the child knows what to expect. It also creates predictability and structure, which, as mentioned earlier in this chapter, are invaluable tools to help improve speed. A sample calendar is shown on the next page.

Visuals can be especially helpful for younger children with slow processing speed. Young children are limited by their language skills, so giving directions verbally (just talking to them) can be doubly hard for young children with slow processing speed. Using picture schedules—a series of pictures that serve as reminders about a sequence of tasks—may prove useful. A sample is shown on page 95.

Jack, a 6-year-old boy with slow processing speed and emerging attention problems, had trouble quickly carrying out and remembering how to complete even simple daily tasks. For instance, in the morning, his parents needed to constantly watch him so that he could get ready for the day (use the toilet, brush teeth, put on clothes already laid out, comb hair). His parents frequently redirected Jack because he was not only a step behind the rest of the family but was also easily distracted. The whole family would run late because Jack always needed extra help, and his parents were feeling run-down and frustrated. They couldn't understand how it could take so long for Jack to complete even the simplest of tasks.

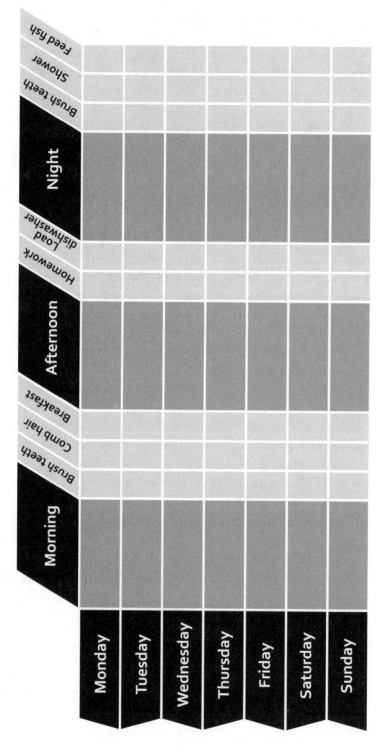

Brush...   **Toilet...**   **Bedtime... zzzzz**

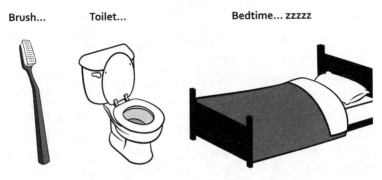

© Semenchenko; © Caraman; © Xpdream | Dreamstime.com

After meeting in our offices, we realized that Jack needed help. It seemed that the strategy of verbally reminding him of daily routines was not enough, so we suggested a picture schedule to help Jack remember important day-to-day tasks such as getting ready in the morning and getting ready for bed. Using these visual aids at home helped to remind Jack of the key steps of daily routines, and ultimately sped Jack up.

Advocate for Your Child at Home

This brings us to the third *A* of the three A's of processing speed: advocate. In later chapters we will discuss how to advocate for your child in other contexts, such as in school and with friends, but here we focus on how to advocate for your child at home. Yes, even in the comforts of their own home, children with slow processing speed often need their parents to act as advocates because they are often described as "lazy," "unmotivated," or "not smart" by family members.

Sometimes parents themselves are not in agreement about their child's difficulties. That is, where one parent could see their child as lazy, the other could see her as having a neuropsychological weakness. Parents may need to help one another understand the true causes, consequences, and realities of their child's slow processing speed. It is best when parents have a similar understanding of the nature of their child's struggles. We know from research that when parents disagree on basic parenting issues, these differences of opinion can lead to inconsistent parenting, confusion, and acting out by the child.

Parents may also be faced with the job of explaining their child's profile to other children in the family. Children with slow processing speed can appear different from their siblings and therefore become the target of teasing. Parents can combat this teasing by helping siblings understand that everyone learns differently and moves at a different pace. We find that parents like to use analogies to explain this idea, such as equating the brain to the processor of a computer. Being slow doesn't mean that the computer doesn't work; it means that the computer just takes a little extra time to load a webpage, download a song, or search on Google for the right information. Parents also find it helpful to point out that everyone has strengths and weaknesses. For instance, although Jack may take longer to get ready for school in the morning, when he's on the soccer field, he's the strongest player on the team—and quicker than anyone else in the family.

Lastly, parents will likely be faced with questions from other family members, friends, and neighbors about their child's slow speed. Why does it take so long for him to get things done? Why does she struggle so much with homework? Can't he hurry up since he's slowing everyone down? These situations can be uncomfortable because you don't always want to explain your child's brain functioning to others.

Some parents prefer to be very forthcoming, explaining that they had their child tested, what the results were, and how slow processing speed is one of the key issues. Others prefer to share less, simply stating, "Jacqueline is smart, but it just takes her a little longer to get things—it's just the way her brain is wired." These short explanations often suffice. As an advocate for your child, you may need to remind others that your child *is not choosing to be slow*. She is not lazy or not smart, nor does she have a behavior problem. She is simply slower at getting things done than other kids her age, and with the right help, will go on to do things just as well as others.

Processing Speed in the Classroom

As hard as it might be for your child to cope with slow processing speed at home, for some kids it's even harder to cope in the classroom. Classrooms run at a certain pace, and when you're slow to keep up, you're going to feel behind. Think about the typical public school classroom: one teacher, an underfunded classroom with 25–30 students, many with unique learning styles. Where does a child with slow processing speed fit into this scenario? Well, a lot depends on the particular teacher. In fact you may already have discovered that some years are much better than others because some teachers seem to "get" your child and your child, in turn, responds well. So why then are some years not as good? Well, like parents, most regular education teachers have never received any training to prepare them for the task of teaching kids with slow processing speed. Even special education teachers don't have much training in this specific area, so what is a parent to do?

In this chapter we attempt to give you some direction, first by helping you identify how your child typically functions in the classroom. Is he anxious, overly relaxed, or always lost? Does he compensate by rushing through, or does he never complete anything? Next, we identify the ideal types of learning environments for these kids. Finally, we identify some specific strategies that have been found to be effective, regardless of the type of learning environment. Teachers and schools have little choice but to think about how to handle kids with slow processing speed. We live in the age of inclusion, and this is a good thing, but it leaves teachers responsible for many special-needs kids. Unfortunately (in our experience) the kids with slow processing speed who don't have behavior problems tend to get lost or literally left behind their peers—and the ones who *do* exhibit significant disruptive behavior problems are sometimes treated unfairly.

What Is the Impact of Slow Processing Speed at School?

Joey, Casey, and Danny were all diagnosed with slow processing speed, yet each one of them functioned and behaved quite differently within the classroom. Joey was just *slow* at everything. At age 8, he was a good reader, but he was having a difficult time getting math facts. He could add, subtract, and multiply, but when his teacher did the "1-minute math" worksheets, he completed the fewest problems of any child in the class. His handwriting was poor, and he resisted writing, so his teacher allowed him to use a computer for writing assignments. His locker and desk were a mess, full of papers that were never handed in, old lunches, and mittens missing their mates. He often appeared as if he wasn't listening or was completely lost in daydreams. Sometimes he would become absorbed in picking at the eczema on his arms or watching the squirrel in the tree. When the teacher gave directions, Joey would sit there picking at his scabs while the other children got out their textbooks and turned to the correct page. Most of the time the teacher ignored Joey—not on purpose, but because he wasn't a problem. He progressed in school, year after year, doing OK but never performing at the level expected of him. By high school, he had the nickname "Mr. Chill," because nothing bothered him—and by *nothing* we really mean nothing! Penalties for missing assignment due dates or showing up late to class— nothing ever seemed to get him anxious enough to do anything on time or well.

Casey had a similar neuropsychological profile to Joey but

was really quite different. Casey's slow processing speed caused him to be anxious about everything. He, like Joey, frequently daydreamed, which caused him to miss what the teacher was saying or what he was supposed to be doing; however, unlike Joey, Casey didn't "chill"; he got anxious. At times he outwardly might look like Joey, sitting quietly at the back of the classroom, but internally he was a mess. His stomach hurt, he obsessed over what he should do, and at times he would cry. Casey tended to get bogged down in details and had trouble distinguishing what was most relevant from minor issues. He was prone to becoming overly emotional about minor or unimportant things, to the point where he would miss the entire point of the assignment. At home he had frequent meltdowns when he would realize that he couldn't get the assignment done on time. He'd scream things such as "I hate you" and "I'm going to kill myself if you make me do this assignment" at his parents, leaving them to wonder if he had an underlying emotional problem. Because of the combination of anxiety and slow processing speed, he had a tendency to shut down quickly on even mildly challenging tasks. Needless to say, this combination made his performance even slower. It is also notable that during the summer, when Casey had no academic demands or issues about performance, he was rarely emotional.

Danny was different from both Joey and Casey. Although slow processing speed was also a major component of Danny's cognitive profile, he didn't cope by becoming anxious or by chilling but by seeming perpetually *lost*. He was the last one of the family out the door in the morning and the last kid out of the classroom in the afternoon. Although Danny was intelligent, few people thought of him as "smart." He rarely initiated conversation, not because he didn't have important things to contribute but because by the time he came up with an answer, the conversation had already moved on. He could read well, but when it came time to write a report on what he'd read, he had no idea where to start. Danny couldn't (or, as his teacher suspected, wouldn't) write a word. He became totally stumped and unable to proceed when confronted with a blank piece of paper. Danny could read the material and seemed to be listening in class, but when it came time to actually participate in class discussions, he seemed at a loss for words.

We find that most of the kids we see with slow processing speed fit into one or more of the categories that Danny, Joey, and Casey illustrate:

• The *chill* kids. These kids tend to take on the persona of the "slow one" and wear it as a badge of honor, to a fault. They know they're not as quick as their friends to do their multiplication tables, and they act as if they don't really care. They'll say things such as "Those kids who do everything on time are just *noobs*." They'll tend to make fun of the kids who win the spelling bees or who always hand in their tests first. When these kids have a teacher who understands them (sometimes the teacher is actually *like* them), they'll have a good year. When they have a teacher who values speed and who views "chilling" as another way of saying *lazy*, they're apt to have a bad school year. Although in some ways it's good to embrace your faults, in the case of these kids, it might be too much of a good thing.

• The *anxious* kids. These kids, like Casey, tend to be nervous all the time. Their already weak processing speed causes them to be anxious, and their anxiety slows them down even further. At home (and sometimes at school) they appear anxious and have meltdowns when presented with tasks they know they can't do. If they have a teacher who understands anxiety and who doesn't put a premium on speed, they'll tend to do well, but a teacher who values quickness and perfection is typically a bad match for this type of child.

• The *lost* kids. These are the kids, like Danny, who are never at the right place at the right time. In high school, they show up in the wrong homeroom on the wrong day, while in elementary school you might find them getting "lost" on the way from the bathroom back to their classroom. Neither anxious nor "chill," these children strike others as more oblivious to their surroundings. Often people will inaccurately assume that they are just not that bright. A teacher who has the time to find the "diamond in the rough" is a perfect match for this type of child. A teacher who is overwhelmed by the demands of the job may promote these kids to the next grade without ever knowing the depth of thought of their capabilities.

Do you recognize any of these characteristics in your child? These are not scientific categories, so your child may not be a perfect match, but you probably notice some commonalities. It's also not that uncommon for kids to act differently at different ages. For example, a "chill" kid may grow up to become an anxious high school student once he knows that he can't fake his way. A kid who spent elementary school "lost" may adopt the persona of a "chilled stoner" because he'd prefer people to think he was "relaxed" instead of "slow" or "not very bright."

So far, we have only alluded to the ideal academic environments for these kids. At the end of the chapter, we give you a list of things that you might find helpful to think about if you have

IS PRIVATE OR PUBLIC EDUCATION BETTER FOR THESE KIDS?

It depends. A public school environment is more than capable of meeting the needs of kids with slow processing speed. And, in fact, public school systems are legally obligated to meet a child's needs. What's more important is the philosophy of the school toward individual learning styles. Most (but not all) private schools have the advantage of small class sizes. This is often a big plus for kids with slow processing speed (actually, it's a plus for almost any kid) because there's less information for them to process and because the teacher has more time available to individualize her approach. We encourage parents to visit possible school environments, keeping in mind some of the points listed on the next couple of pages.

an option of pairing your child with the right teacher. But overall, there are some general points to keep in mind with regard to finding the right environment.

Ideal Academic Environments for Kids with Slow Processing Speed: The Teacher

Ideally, all children should have an academic environment perfectly fitted for them. This isn't possible, although we see parents all the time who think it should (or even could) be. That doesn't mean you shouldn't know what the ideal is. We frequently tell parents that gifted teachers don't need our suggestions because they are usually already doing what we suggest. You might find yourself in the best school district in the best school building with all the best bells and whistles, but if your child's teacher is a bad match, none of the rest of it matters. Conversely, a gifted teacher can work in any situation with almost any kind of obstacle and still make learning exciting. So what makes a gifted teacher for kids with slow processing speed? We've found there are a few traits that are particularly important.

EMPATHY

Good teachers tend to be *empathic,* and it's really important for children with slow processing speed to have teachers who can empathize with their difficulties. To be able to do that, teachers have to be *willing to learn about the child's unique difficulties.* Getting a formal evaluation can be a good place to start educating your child's teacher about his difficulties as even the most empathic teacher may find it hard to empathize with something she doesn't understand. When presented with test data that document a student's profile (see Chapter 9 for examples), it usually becomes crystal clear to teachers what the problem is, and this new clarity often starts them on the road to remediation and accommodation.

SENSE OF HUMOR

Kids with slow processing speed also tend to respond well to teachers who have a *good sense of humor.* Overly serious teachers can be quite good at motivating certain types of students, but it tends to make these kids more nervous. (Again, keep in mind that *good* teachers, regardless of their personality, tend to do well with these students—even the more serious teachers.) Teachers with a good sense of humor tend to have a better ability to *change tempo* when it's needed. In other words, when plans go awry in the classroom or when it's obvious the lesson is reaching different kids at different times, these teachers have the ability to change their presentation style or the pace of the instruction. Their instruction shifts to reflect the needs of the students in the class. They also tend to *not expect a quick fix.* They realize these issues are not fixable in a day or in a year. In fact, they may think they're not worthy of "fixing" at all, since these types of teachers tend to appreciate all types of learning styles. They know that although the child may look like she is choosing to move in slow motion, nothing could be further from the truth.

THOUGHTFUL ABOUT WORKLOAD

In terms of the workload, the best teachers for kids with slow processing speed tend to:

- Deemphasize busy work.

- Show a willingness to adjust homework assignments to "fit" with a student's pace.

- Balance the common needs of all the students with the specific needs of individual students.

- Be excited by the use of technology in their classrooms because it makes it easier to adapt instruction.

- Be both organized and flexible.

These teachers understand that not everyone learns at the same pace, and they are willing to practice what they preach by adapting assignments so that all the kids are appropriately challenged. Overly organized teachers tend to drive these kids crazy because their slow speed tends to mess up the teachers' well-

---

"I'm a teacher reading this book. What advice would you give me?" Rather than giving advice, we'd prefer to give you some questions that are important to consider. As we've indicated above, these kids can manifest their difficulties very differently, and therefore it's best to think about the factors in the learning and teaching process that are important for these kids. Ask yourself:

- "Am I creating an environment in which this child's learning style is valued?"
- "Am I creating an environment that maximizes the child's attentional skills so as to maximize the speed at which she is able to perform?"
- "Are the students given ample opportunities to practice skills (so that they become more fluent with the task) while minimizing busy work (that can slow down the process)?"
- "Are the students given the opportunity to learn skills to the point where they feel comfortable and know something automatically?"
- "Are the new skills and knowledge presented at a rate and amount that allow students time to learn and in a manner that gives them enough information yet does not overload them?"
- "Am I maximizing their processing speed by getting them to think about what they already know about a skill or topic, and are they given the opportunity to build upon that information in an organized fashion?"

organized plans. Conversely, overly flexible teachers tend to overlook the fact that these kids need some amount of rigidity so that they can work within certain parameters. The perfect teacher displays a combination of the two.

School Characteristics

From reading the previous section you might think that it's all about the teacher, but of course the role of the school is also key. What are the ingredients that can make school more successful for these kids?

PARENT–TEACHER COLLABORATION

First and foremost, the school has to provide an environment *open to parent–teacher collaboration.* In fact, the school should be willing to collaborate on many levels—not only with parents but with occupational therapists, counselors, neuropsychologists, and any other personnel who may be involved in your child's care.

ATTENTION TO INDIVIDUAL DIFFERENCES

Second, there needs to be an environment that conveys a *positive emphasis on individual differences,* where different learning styles are valued, and an emphasis on a *social curriculum,* wherein students' emotional and social needs are valued, not only their academic needs. Along with this emphasis comes a *school that promotes kindness and tolerance of differences.* Yes, almost every school says it values differences, but the school actually has to *show* it by identifying strengths while supporting disabilities and empowering students.

LACK OF CLUTTER

Kids with slow processing speed tend to respond best in a *school that is neat, clean, and uncluttered, both physically and visually.* Does that mean that they can't learn in a classroom or school that is filled to the ceiling with interesting materials? No, but they tend to respond better when there is less to process in the environment.

RECESS

These children also need down time, and schools that provide multiple *recess periods* during the day can be a wonderful way for kids with slow processing speed to recharge and maintain their focus.

"What about specific types of academic environments, such as Montessori or Waldorf schools?" There are a number of different academic environments, any of which might be the right fit for your child. Montessori and Waldorf are two of the more popular private school environments, and both have their benefits and liabilities for kids with slow processing speed. For the right child, Montessori can be wonderful. It is an individually driven curriculum, and for kids who run on a slower speed, the slower pace of the classroom can be perfect; however, kids who have significant attention and organizational issues can find this environment challenging because it is relatively unstructured. A Waldorf curriculum places much less emphasis on the individual pace of the learner, but it does place great value on active learning, a depth of instruction (in contrast to a fast-paced curriculum), and the importance of movement and recess. Either one of these environments can work, but it really depends on the child. The best advice is to seek the guidance of the school personnel. Be honest with the school if you have knowledge of your child's learning style and let them help you decide whether it's a good fit or not.

FLEXIBLE GROUPING OF STUDENTS

These kids tend to respond best when there are flexible groupings of students—or, at the very least, thoughtful groupings of
students. In other words, they do better when there are kids with
different "speeds" in different groups, all bringing their own
expertise to the project.

Specific Strategies and Accommodations

The list of specific educational strategies for kids with slow processing speed is potentially endless, in part because there isn't
a "one-size-fits-all" strategy. Having slow processing speed isn't
like having dyslexia, for which we can recommend documented
treatments that have been found to be effective. Instead, it's a
lot of trial and error, using strategies that have been found to
be effective for kids with all sorts of executive dysfunction. That
being said, there are some factors that we've found particularly
effective for these kids, each of which is elaborated below.

AMPLE TIME . . . AND TIME MANAGEMENT

The most obvious, and most important, strategy within the classroom is to *allow ample time* to get things done. Even if your child
can figure out what might be a good plan (and particularly if he
can't), many situations in the classroom don't afford the necessary
time to get it done. Giving the child more time is key, whether it's
a project, an exam, or a standardized test such as the SAT or
ACT. But sometimes extra time isn't feasible, and in those cases
children need to have coping strategies such as remaining calm,
asking for help, and speaking up.

As kids grow into adolescents, they should start to be able to
verbalize their difficulties by saying things such as "It sometimes
takes me a long time to come up with an answer. Give me a little
more time so that I can think about this and I'll get back to you."
At the same time, extra time shouldn't be another word for *stall-*

ing, as sometimes kids will use the extra time as a way to delay the task or to get out of a stressful situation. They need to learn the difference between "extra time to get it done right" and "not using the extra time wisely."

Along with extra time is teaching a child to manage time, as these kids not only tend to be slower than average but also tend to:

- Be late with projects, even when given ample time, because they haven't learned how to keep track of time.

- Feel pressured by any time constraints (even ones that are appropriate), which cause them to feel anxious.

- Misjudge time in that they have no idea how long something will take, how long it takes the average person to do something versus how long it will take them, and how much time is left to do something.

Given these points, it's clearly important that kids learn to tell time. This may seem obvious, but we find that kids with slow processing speed often have other difficulties (learning disabilities, ADHD) that make it tough for them to learn to tell time. Thus they need specific teaching of telling time because they generally don't pick up this concept on their own. This is true not just for the time of day but also for the time of year. They have difficulty learning the days of the week and months of the year and have trouble knowing how far away Christmas is when it's August. Teaching the time using a clock or watch with hands can be better than a digital clock because they can actually "see" the time moving. Similarly, keeping a calendar in the classroom and referring to it frequently is a good way to help them to measure the passage of time.

Kids with slow processing speed tend to be chronically late to class, due in part to their being "lost" or "chilling" or even losing track of where they are, but it's also often a product of the fact that they have no concept of how long it can take them to get from point A to point B. They don't know how long it takes them to unlock their locker, restock their backpack, and get to their history class at the other end of the school. When they get to class late, the teacher understandably thinks that they were trying to avoid class or didn't care, but the opposite can be true. In fact, the child can be completely surprised when he arrives in class 5 minutes late.

This kind of behavior won't likely be fixed without clear, focused teaching about what is wrong (the management of time) and how to fix it (strategies for getting to their locker and class on time). The plan will need to address the actual problem with getting to class (this could be a host of things) and then a detailed plan for how to fix it. Most important, *the child will need to practice the plan many times* if there is any hope for change. The biggest problem with these kids and their relation to time is that they are often not given a chance to learn the skill to the point of automaticity. Someone will hand them a calendar, for example, and show them how to put one week's assignments on it or show them once how to get to class quickly—without then guiding them to overlearn these skills. They have to have repeated practice to have any chance of change. In terms of keeping a calendar, it means having daily checkpoints for months, perhaps even years, before they internalize its use. For getting to class on time, it may mean monitoring the child for a month before a timely walk from point A to point B becomes automatic. Lastly, when the schedule changes, you can't expect these children to automatically transfer the skills to their new schedule. Be prepared to support these kids for many years—while holding on to the knowledge that it will pay off in years to come.

In addition to time management strategies, there are a number of more specific strategies that tend to help kids with slow processing speed. For example:

KEEPING A SECOND SET OF TEXTBOOKS AT HOME

Not having to lug textbooks back and forth to school (and get them in and out of the locker and backpack) is a real time-saver for these kids. If possible, there should be a set of textbooks at school that they can use and a separate set at home that can stay there until the end of the year.

AVAILABILITY OF TECHNOLOGY

In general, technology can be a real time-saver for these kids, especially if it limits how much work has to be handwritten and facilitates homework transfer from home to school. Being able to complete assignments on the computer is generally much faster than handwriting. It also helps in communicating with teachers. Sometimes these kids don't know that they're behind until long after class. Having the opportunity to correspond with their teachers by e-mail, after class is over and when they've had time to think about what they need, can be much preferable to feeling like they need to ask everything during class.

One caveat to this is when kids are required to interface with multiple teachers on multiple websites. These kids do much better when schools have a single website for all teachers and assignments than when teachers are allowed to have their own websites. It can be paralyzing for a 10th-grade student at 9:00 P.M. when she is trying to check six different teachers' websites, all located on different servers. In that case, technology is a time-waster, not a time-saver.

MODELS OF THE FINISHED PRODUCT OF ASSIGNMENTS

Kids with slow processing speed benefit greatly from being able to review what a finished assignment looks like before they do their own. Because these students tend to have problems seeing the big picture, showing them the big picture at the outset can be very helpful. Even more helpful is having them estimate the time that it would take them to complete portions of the assignment.

EXPLICIT BEGINNING AND END POINTS FOR ASSIGNMENTS

It is helpful for children with slow processing speed to know exactly where to start when beginning assignments—and also knowing when to stop. For instance, in the case of younger children, this may mean setting a time limit for homework (for example, 30 minutes a night). For older children, chunking a reading assignment into sections is more helpful than giving a vague assignment (for example, explicitly stating "Read Chapters 1 through 3 by next Wednesday" versus "Start reading the book by next Wednesday").

"WHAT CAN PARENTS DO TO BE HELPFUL TO TEACHERS?"

Throughout this chapter, we've talked about what schools and teachers can do for these kids, but parents play a large role too. Our biggest recommendation is to know that you're part of a team and, to the best extent that you can, to collaborate with the teachers and school. Try not to become an adversary. When you find yourself in the role of adversary (and many parents unfortunately find themselves in this role), one of the best ways to move from an adversarial role to a collaborative role is to get more information. Have your child evaluated either by the school or privately. Become more knowledgeable about the school's curriculum so that you can think about whether it's right for your child. Become aware of your beliefs and attitudes about the school and teacher(s); if you're negative, this will affect the attitudes of your child, your child's teacher, and the school's administrator.

PRACTICAL STRATEGIES FOR ACCOMMODATING SLOW PROCESSING SPEED AT SCHOOL

- *Advocate for your child to have ample—often extra—time.*
    - This may mean extra time on exams, standardized tests, and homework assignments.
    - It does *not* mean making it possible for the child to stall.
    - Teach your child to advocate for extra time for himself as he gets older.
- *Teach time management.*
    - Teach your child to tell time.
    - Make sure plans for getting around school and completing homework on schedule are practiced to the point of being overlearned.
- *Keep an extra set of textbooks at home.*
- *Take advantage of technology as a time-saver.*
    - Make sure your child can minimize handwriting by using a computer to complete assignments when possible.
    - Have the child communicate with teachers by e-mail at home or using portals set up by the school.
    - Avoid the computer for teacher communication if your child would have to contact each teacher individually.
- *Ask for examples of completed homework for your child to review before doing the assignment.*
- *Make sure assignments are clearly structured and uncluttered:*
    - Clear beginning and end points
    - No redundancy
    - Simple, uncluttered visuals
- *Avoid multitasking.*
    - Ask for alternatives to note taking during lectures.

HOMEWORK THAT IS NEITHER REDUNDANT NOR CLUTTERED

Worksheets should not be visually overwhelming and confusing. Kids with slow processing speed don't need to waste precious time doing the same types of problems over and over again once they've learned the concept. Similarly, too much information or too many problems on one worksheet may look overwhelming to them, and they may shut down as a result.

REDUCED NEED FOR MULTITASKING

Multitasking can be overwhelming and can slow down the whole process. In older students the biggest example of multitasking is the need to take notes while listening to lectures. Thus, we recommend *assistance with note taking* by getting the notes in advance, getting an outline, or getting an audio recording and listening to the lecture later.

Pulling It All Together: The Three A's of Processing Speed in the Classroom

Remember *accept, accommodate,* and *advocate,* our three A's of processing speed? Well, they are important in school too.

ACCEPTANCE

The first step toward reaching acceptance is getting a thorough evaluation from either the school or an independent practitioner. Without a thorough evaluation that documents the problem(s), it's hard for teachers to actually accept that your child has a problem. The test data can be crucial in helping the teachers understand the underlying issues and accepting the accommodations.

But teachers aren't the only ones who need to "accept"— parents do too. You may find that it's relatively easy to accept your child's slower pace at home but that when it comes to school tasks, you have absolutely no tolerance for slowness. You may be able to live with the fact that your son is the last one in the family to make a decision about what cereal she wants for breakfast, but you can't tolerate the fact that she can't finish writing 10 sentences for her weekly spelling words within a 2-hour time frame.

"I have accepted the fact that my child needs tutoring, but he doesn't want it. What do I do?" If you've accepted the fact, you are halfway there, so don't give up hope. It's pretty common for kids with learning issues to resist tutoring. There are a couple of reasons for this resistance. First, many times these kids have had some kind of tutoring or remediation in the past and it didn't work—or it was really hard work—and they didn't reap the benefits. Thus, they are reluctant to try it again. Second, the fact that they need some kind of tutoring or homework support brings them face to face with the fact that they have a disability, and when the disability is "processing speed problems" and no one really knows exactly what will fix them, it can be tough for them to accept.

Sharing some of the information you've learned in this book can be a way to begin to help your child accept her disabilities. Having the school psychologist or the professional who documented the processing speed deficits share the results from the evaluation, and what they mean, with your child is also a great idea. In addition, it's very important to find the right tutor. How do you know someone is the right tutor? Your child will be glad to see him. A good tutor will make your child's life easier. It may take a while, but if it's taking months and you're not seeing results and your child doesn't like the tutor, it's probably time to find a new tutor. So, our suggestions are: *Make sure you and your child accept the fact that tutoring can work, make your child part of the decision-making process with regard to picking the right tutor,* and *let your child know that if the tutor doesn't make his life easier, you'll find a tutor who does.*

Homework incompletion, or time to completion, may just be the most difficult thing for parents to accept. It may very well be what makes your life miserable through the school year. Accepting this is something that is hard for your child—and remembering it on a daily (sometimes momentary) basis is key. That is not an excuse, however, for getting your child off the hook. It is instead the first step in accepting that he will need help, whether it's in the form of the suggestions we've listed above, getting a tutor to help with homework, or finding a way to build more homework time into your family's schedule. If you can accept that homework is a problem that can't be controlled by yelling or wishing, then you can accept that there are solutions and you might be ready to give them a try.

ACCOMMODATING

In terms of accommodating at school, much of this chapter has offered suggestions for appropriate accommodations. Extra time is key for nearly every child with slow processing speed, but other accommodations are likely also warranted. Work with your school and your child's teacher to come up with a plan—either a formalized one such as an IEP or a less formal plan if an IEP is not warranted.

ADVOCATING

Lastly, advocating can be one of the most important roles you can have as a parent. You may find yourself in the unlikely position of having to educate your child's teacher about his disability, and you may find yourself fighting with the school for appropriate services. Some parents relish this role, whereas others find it far out of their comfort zone. In the early elementary years, it is an important role for parents to play, particularly if there is a lack of understanding on the part of the teachers or school. If you do find yourself in the role of the crusading advocate, it's our advice to approach the school as a collaborative partner. Keep your child's best interests in mind. We find that sometimes parents get into power struggles with the school, and although there are times when that is the right approach, most of the time it isn't.

Good advocates don't fight first; they leave fighting as a last option. Our advice would be to do the same, because one day your child will need to advocate for herself. She'll be a high school or college student, and she'll have learned how to advocate by watching what you did. If she sees you constantly fighting with her teachers, she might become a college student who will be needlessly arguing with professors about accommodations they may have been quite willing to make. On the other hand, if she never sees you stand up for her, she may be the college student who never even asks for appropriate accommodations.

Managing a child with slow processing speed at school is challenging for all involved—teachers, parents, and students. However, by using the strategies in this chapter and thinking as a collaborator with school personnel, we hope that you and your child can focus on the opportunities for accomplishment that the learning environment provides. Your child's performance at school sets the stage for the way he will cope with challenges in life. Finding the right balance of accommodating the challenges versus accepting them is tough, but it can be done. Take advantage of the support offered at school, do everything you can to find the best academic environment, and remember that homework isn't everything.

seven

Processing Speed and Social Relationships

Nathan's parents were worried. It was the end of fifth grade, and he hadn't gotten invited to one birthday party all year long. Now it was June, the end-of-school-year party was next week, and Nathan didn't want to go. He had felt left out all year and was confused as to why. His parents were too and decided to speak to his teacher, Ms. Brayson, who they hoped could shed some light on why Nathan was on the social fringe of his class. Ms. Brayson was actually surprised to hear that Nathan had never been invited to parties because he seemed to be well liked by his peers or, as Ms. Brayson noted, "He's definitely not disliked by his peers." Ms. Brayson did, however, describe Nathan as often being in "dreamland" during class, saying that that led him to being slow at picking up on jokes and sarcasm. She didn't realize that might result in his not being invited to playdates. After all, Nathan had a reading disability, and although his profile was also significant for slow processing speed, he didn't have true social problems. So how could it be that he was never invited to parties?

Although we don't tend to think of processing speed as a necessary part of social relationships, Nathan's story shows that it can play a role in a number of ways, some of them subtle or operating beneath the surface of interactions. In fact, though, there is a big association between processing speed and social skills.

Part of this association exists because many children with slow processing speed have other syndromes, such as ADHD and the autism spectrum disorders, in which social problems are common. However, our research has shown that this is not the whole story.

Regardless of any diagnosis, children with slow processing speed are at greater risk for social deficits. They have higher rates of social and language delays in early childhood. For instance, in the sample of nearly 600 children seen in our clinic, we found that of those children with slow processing speed, over *one-third* had experienced social difficulties before the age of 5 (for example, problems approaching other children to play, trouble with to-and-fro activities). We also found that nearly *half* of children with slow processing speed had some problems with communication in early childhood (for example, being slow to talk). This combination of slow processing speed and language delays is a recipe for social problems at an early age.

Not only do many children with slow processing speed show early social delays, but many continue to have social skills problems throughout their development. In our sample, 52% of the children with slow processing speed were reported by their parents to have *current* social difficulties. The most frequently reported problems were difficulties with social communication (for example, having an easy to-and-fro conversation: 51%), social awareness (for example, picking up on social cues from a peer: 54%), and social cognition (for example, being on the same "wavelength" as their peers: 50%). Teachers often see similar problems in the school environment, with 50% of the students with slow processing speed in our sample displaying social problems in the school environment. These problems included things such as difficulty spontaneously complimenting others, problems quickly picking up on social cues from peers, and a reluctance to join group activities.

The social difficulties seen in our sample of children with slow processing speed were usually *mild to moderate,* meaning that their social problems might be apparent only in certain situations (for example, in an overwhelming or fast-paced social interaction) and are likely responsive to some general supports from parents and teachers (for example, getting help from a parent to set up a playdate with a friend). Only a small percentage (7%) of the children in our sample showed *severe* social problems, such as not wanting to play with others at all or having no close friendships. This small group of children with severe social problems often had problems beyond slow processing speed, such as having a developmental disorder (for example, autism) or psychiatric difficulties (for example, severe depression).

We should point out that not every child with slow processing speed has problems with social skills, and the impairment can vary greatly. The list on the next page outlines some of the ways that slow processing speed impacts social relationships. It's not that kids with slow processing speed have poor social skills per se; it's that their slow rate of processing causes problems in daily life that make social relationships more problematic.

For instance, Jacob was a very empathic child who could pick up on social cues at a very mature level—*if* he was given adequate time to think through a situation. He had no problem understanding the concept of social relationships, but he often missed social opportunities because he didn't respond quickly enough to someone's question or social overture. His teacher described him as a kid "on the periphery" who was frequently noted to walk around the perimeter of the playground before he settled into a game during recess. Unfortunately, by the time he decided what activity he wanted to participate in, the game was already in full gear, and the kids who were playing often didn't want to change the teams to accommodate him. It's not that they didn't like him or wouldn't have wanted him to play with them. He was just too late to be a part of it. Sometimes it took him so long to decide what he wanted to do that recess was already over before he made up his mind.

Similarly, Seth's parents were worried because he complained that no one played with him at recess, and so they asked his teacher to formally observe him on the playground. She explained to them that recess was only 10–15 minutes long and that for the first 5 minutes of recess Seth was fussing with the zipper on his

HOW DOES SLOW PROCESSING SPEED AFFECT A CHILD'S FRIENDSHIPS?

Slow processing speed can affect social relationship in general and friendships in particular in many different ways. Some of the more common issues include the following:

- Children with slow processing speed take longer to pick up on social cues in general, thus missing the point of the social exchange.
- Interactions can seem stilted or awkward because it takes them a long time to figure out a response.
- They lose track of what's happening during pretend play or games, causing their peers to become frustrated with them.
- They are disorganized in relaying stories or reporting events, causing peers to lose interest in what they are saying.
- Poor time management (for example, always running late) causes friends to become exasperated with them and generally gets in the way of positive relationships.
- Reactions to jokes and sarcasm can be just a few seconds behind, which can make them seem a bit "off" to their peers.
- Slow work performance makes it difficult when working with a group and on group assignments.

coat and his shoelaces, which had been untied all day because he didn't have time to tie them (yes, it took him a long time to tie his laces). The next 5 minutes of recess he spent slowly perusing what everyone else was doing. When the 2-minute warning bell sounded for the kids to start to wrap up their games and come inside, Seth had just asked the kids who were playing soccer if he could join them. They mostly ignored him since they were trying to finish their game, although one of his friends said, "Why didn't you get over here sooner? We needed another player!"

As kids grow into adolescence, the pace of social relationships gets even quicker. Kids relate to each other in short bursts of information. In high school, social plans are often negotiated in the 3 or 4 minutes between classes. If your child is the kind of teen who takes a very long time to open his locker, get out the right books, and walk down the hall to the classroom, he may be missing out on the possibility of being invited to someone's party or making plans to go to the movie with friends. It's not that his friends didn't want him to join them; it's just that he wasn't there when they made their plans and they (like most adolescents) don't think about who should have been invited. Parents may hear these stories and think that their child has problems with social skills—and sometimes, as in the case of a child with a pervasive developmental disorder, it might be true; however, it's often just the effect of slow processing speed.

Naturally, parents want to help their child or teenager learn to be better at social relationships. But how do they go about doing that in this case? First of all, if your child has a documented disability such as autism or an autism spectrum disorder, more than just slow processing speed is at play here and you should avail yourself of any and all programs, such as social skills training, applied behavior analysis (ABA), or relationship development intervention (RDI), that target your child's underlying weakness. Second, regardless of whether processing speed is your child's primary problem or an associated problem, there are things you can do that will help her *accept* her potential limitations, *accommodate* her issues, and learn to *advocate* for herself in social situations.

The Three A's of Processing Speed and Friendships

ACCEPTANCE

As we mentioned earlier, emerging research, including that from our own clinic, has shown that children with slow processing speed are at high risk for social problems. They often have difficulty initiating or sustaining conversations in a timely manner. It can take them a long time to communicate their ideas, feelings, and needs because it can take a significant amount of time to organize their thoughts. Although they are more than capable of understanding and interpreting verbal and nonverbal cues, they often have difficulty paying attention to social cues and interpreting them in "real time." This can result in a cycle of what we consider "social neglect," which can then lead to social withdrawal and isolation.

Knowing that social problems are a possible area of concern is the first step in fixing the problem. But keep in mind that it's important not to "overinterpret" these social problems, meaning it's important not to jump to conclusions that your child's problems are due to something more significant, such as autism or severe depression. We have assessed many children whose parents have run from doctor to doctor, asking questions such as "Is the reason my child doesn't get invited to parties that he's autistic?" or "Does my child not play with kids on the playground because she's depressed or anxious?" When the doctors give them the information that their child isn't autistic or suicidal, they are sometimes disappointed because they want to know the cause of the problem. Since processing speed wasn't assessed in the course of an interview with a doctor, they are left with no answers to their questions. This is why a thorough evaluation with formal testing can be so crucial—even when the primary issue relates to social skills. Ruling out other causes, or getting to the root of the problem, is the absolute first crucial step in accepting the problem.

A thorough assessment, such as that provided in a comprehensive neuropsychological evaluation, should include an assessment of a child's ability to learn and practice social skills in a variety of environments—at school, home, and out in the world. A child has to be able to adequately process and express what is seen and heard and then respond appropriately. Knowing whether your child has problems with auditory or visual processing (or both) will allow you to know where and when to accept his limitations. A good evaluation should identify the strengths and weaknesses of a child's social behavior, ideally by observing the student during peer interactions, but more often (due to time and cost) through teacher and parent reports. If your child struggles with slow processing speed and you are worried about social deficits, the types of problems to take notice of include the following:

- Appearing to have difficulty sustaining attention during social interactions

- Taking a long time to understand/grasp social concepts

- Seeming not to be listening to you

- Being unable to quickly "roll with the punches" of complex social situations

- Failing to respond to peers who try to initiate conversations

- Having difficulty with word retrieval, which results in trouble answering questions

- "Missing a beat" when it comes to responding to questions, laughing at jokes, or understanding sarcasm

- Needing more time to respond in social interactions or conversations. This is particularly true when the conversation is emotionally charged.

- Missing out on social opportunities because he was just too late to get the invitation or respond to the invitation

One important point to keep in mind is that even though you might expect these issues—and should accept that they may be present and outside of your child's control—that isn't the end of the story. In fact, there are many ways to accommodate and even treat these problematic behaviors.

ACCOMMODATING

There are numerous ways to accommodate the social skills deficits seen in kids with slow processing speed. Not all of them will be necessary for your child, and some may be more relevant at different times in development. The more common recommendations we make include the following suggestions.

Simplify Social Situations and Provide Guidance

One of the more important—and obvious—accommodations is to allow your child more time to process social interactions. If your child is young, the best way to do that is by limiting the number of students with whom your child interacts or by controlling the environment. For instance, you can schedule only one playmate/friend at a time to decrease the need to process and respond quickly to complex social interactions. It can be particularly helpful, when planning playdates, to select a peer with similar interests. During playdates stay in close proximity (as much as is developmentally appropriate for your child's age) so that you can facilitate interactions (for younger children) or offer hints after the fact on how the child could have interacted more successfully. It can be most helpful to identify one or two major behaviors that you've noticed are causing trouble with friends and work on those. In giving this feedback, you want to make sure that your comments are gentle and loving but not too subtle. For example, avoid putdowns such as "You didn't listen at all to your friend. That was rude." Instead, it's more helpful to say something like this:

> "When your friend was talking really fast about the Lego spaceship he wanted to build, you seemed to not be listening, but I know you were interested in what he had to say. I'm wondering if it was just hard for you to process what he was saying because he was talking so fast. Next time, ask him to speak more slowly."

When children hit the preteen years, it's much more difficult to control their social relationships and to be available to provide this type of concrete feedback. Thus, you may need to look for teachable moments when you can talk about the child's day and help her deconstruct what might have gone wrong. Teach your child about her learning profile so that she can begin to notice when slow processing speed might be causing her difficulty, as well as knowing how to capitalize on her own strengths. Some of the best ways of helping children accommodate for their weak processing speed include the following suggestions:

- Teach them appropriate ways to slow down the environment by asking people to speak more slowly or saying things such as "Give me a second, because I need time to think about that."

- Teach appropriate ways to ask for clarification, such as "What did you mean when you said that?" or "I didn't get everything that you said. Can you say it one more time?"

- Limit the number of peers with whom your child interacts, because the smaller the group, the less to process. Even in the teen years parents can have some influence over this decision.

- Teach your child ways of getting more involved in the pace of the conversation by nodding when someone is speaking or saying things such as "That's interesting" or "I understand" or even just "Uh-huh."

- Make sure they look at and focus on the individual who is talking. Observing someone more closely adds another sensory input and can help facilitate the processing of information.

- Teach your child to be an active listener who becomes adept at interpreting the underlying feelings being expressed by the person's tone of voice, facial expressions, and body language. If the speed of the verbal information is too fast, these additional cues can help the child understand what is being conveyed.

As you can see from this list, many of these items are things that can be taught to your child, but you can't just sit him down with a list and expect these sorts of things to be learned in a day or even a year. Instead these are things that you should keep in mind as you observe and parent your child. Our advice is to wait for teachable moments that lend themselves to discussion. Sometimes this will be after you've observed the child with other kids. Other times it may be when your child comes to you and says "No one likes me" or "I'm never included in games on the playground."

At these moments, your first job is to listen with an ear toward empathy and another toward analyzing what is happening. Sometimes empathy is enough, and it may be all your child really wants at the time. Other times, she might be open to one or maybe two suggestions about behaviors that may be getting in her way. For example:

> "When people talk, you seem to tune them out if they're talking too fast. Try suggesting that they slow down. Be sure to look at them when they're talking to you because sometimes I notice that you start looking around the room when the conversation moves too fast and it causes you to stop listening to what they're saying."

Don't overwhelm your child with all the negatives at one time. Over time, though, share tips such as these:

- "Make sure to ask your teacher for clarification when you don't understand the assignment."

- "Try being more active when you're listening to someone by nodding your head and making eye contact."

- "Ask questions and paraphrase what was said so that you're sure you heard it correctly."

Scaffold Social Interactions

Not only can you simplify social interactions and provide specific suggestions for your child, but you can also set up the social interactions in a way that provides scaffolding for him. By *scaffolding* we mean gently helping your child out in difficult social situations and then slowly stepping out of the interaction so that your child can manage things on his own. For instance, setting up a playdate for your 6-year-old son with slow processing speed won't necessarily guarantee a good day. When your son's friend arrives, your child might be happy to see him but at a loss as to what to do next. Coming up with ideas for activities and getting play started is hard for children with slow processing speed, especially young children. As a parent, you might need to get creative by helping your child set up activities, such as a finger painting station or a Lego building project, before his friend arrives. Once the friend gets there, you may need to stay close for the first 10 minutes to help your child get situated and assist him in figuring out ideas for what he and his friend can do. For instance, you can say things such as "Maybe you guys can build a new city on the moon and I'll come back in a bit and you can tell me all about it."

In addition to scaffolding the initial exchanges between your child and her friends, you can provide in-the-moment scaffolding by modeling how to ask a good question by saying, for example, "Katie, what else did you do this weekend?" Even teenagers benefit from seeing these types of questions modeled. They also may need scaffolding to help get a plan going. If it's a social outing, you may need to help your teen brainstorm some possible activities, offer to help drop off and pick up so that you can subtly help structure the timing of the activity, or assist her in getting ready so that she won't be late and disappoint her friends.

Provide Support for Organization and Communication

In addition to these general interventions, kids with slow processing speed often need help *organizing their thoughts* so that they can communicate better. They frequently have difficulty expressing themselves clearly and concisely and may make comments that are poorly organized and sequenced. Their frequent problems with quick word retrieval and verbal organization cause them to "talk around" a subject and make it difficult for the listener to know what they're trying to say. Sometimes their social conversations may seem disconnected and tangential, and their speech may be peppered with ambiguous words such as "thingy" or "that stuff" or "You know what I mean—that thingamadoodle." If this is a problem for your child, some of the following suggestions might be helpful:

- When you go to the movies or watch a TV show together, spend some time afterward discussing the story by describing the plot of the movie from start to finish. Limit your child's comments to the important information. If he starts to veer off topic, pull him back by focusing on the chronological telling of the story itself. This approach can also be used to help your child talk about experiences more effectively. For example, if he had a great day at school, have him call a grandparent to tell about the experience, but first practice it with an ear toward sequence and organization.

- Video-record your child on your cell phone while she is telling you a story and then evaluate the sequence and organization.

- Have your child explain a video game to a sibling or friend who doesn't know how to play.

- Help your child understand which information is primary and which is secondary.

- Help your child focus on the "big picture" of the story so that organization can flow from large topic to smaller ones.

- Get the child comfortable using words such as *first, second*, and *third* when explaining a topic. If your child is having trouble relating an experience, give her cues such as

"What happened first?" and "And then what happened?" and "What happened last?" Make sure to give her time to come up with a response before asking her another question.

- When your child is relaying a story that you can't follow, don't just nod and pretend to listen (as most parents have done once or twice). Make sure to be an active listener who says things such as "I couldn't follow what you were saying."

- Pictures can be a great way to help children organize a story, particularly stories such as their day at the zoo or their latest vacation.

- Use cooking as a way to help teach verbal organization skills. For instance, have your child learn and articulate the steps it takes to make cookies and teach them to a friend.

Provide Assistance during Complex and Fast-Paced Situations

Finally, it's worth mentioning again that kids with slow processing speed have the most difficulty when confronted with *complex, unfamiliar, fast-paced social situations*. These types of situations can occur anywhere and anytime, but they are very frequently present in sports. For this reason sports can sometimes be problematic for these kids. But that shouldn't exclude them from participating. In the box on pages 130–131, we offer some help with negotiating the world of sports if your child has slow processing speed. Other suggestions to keep in mind when the situations are new and complicated include the following:

- Help your child learn to notice when social situations start to feel complicated. Rather than putting pressure on him to "keep up the pace," teach him to consciously observe and learn to slow down.

- Recognize when emotions or the situation is becoming

USING SPORTS AS A WAY TO PROMOTE SOCIAL SKILLS IN KIDS WITH SLOW PROCESSING SPEED

Organized sports are a great way to enhance social relationships, but sometimes sports can be especially challenging for kids with slow processing speed—even for kids who are athletically inclined. Although it's hard to provide hard-and-fast rules to support your child during sporting activities, here are some points to keep in mind:

- Kids with slow processing speed sometimes (but definitely not always) prefer more noncompetitive sports such as martial arts, swimming, horseback riding, or biking because the speed aspect of some sports can be overwhelming. If that's the case, help your child choose an appropriate activity.

- Take into account your child's interests and ability levels and choose a team that accommodates her skill and processing speed level.

- If competition is difficult for your child to handle, interview the coach and assess the league to make sure it's not too competitive.

- Selecting a team or sport where the focus is on teaching and practicing the skills needed to play the game provides a child with slow processing speed more time to practice, which can lead to quicker processing speed when it's time to actually play the game.

- Practice skills with your child at home so that the skills become more automatic (for example, throwing, catching, dribbling, or shooting a basketball).

- Make sure it's a team or sport where good sportsmanship is not just encouraged but also taught and practiced (emphasis on teamwork as opposed to only quick-

> ness, complimenting other players, knowing when it's appropriate to play aggressively and when it's not).
>
> • Be sure the coach offers positive reinforcement for trying and does not criticize or stress mistakes. It can also be a good idea to talk to the coach about your child's issue if you think it could be a significant problem.
>
> • Try not to be that typical "poor sportsmanship parent": the one who yells and screams on the sidelines during practices and games. It's generally stressful for all kids to see their parents getting worked up on the sidelines during games, but it's particularly stressful for kids with slow processing speed. Hearing their parents yelling commands from the sidelines, or worse, yelling at the coach or ref, only serves to add stress to what might already be a stressful situation.

overly intense so that your child can shift to a more positive and calm environment when possible.

• Prepare your child in advance if you know that the situation has the potential to be overwhelming. Review what will happen and who will be there. If it's a situation where the child will be seeing people she hasn't seen in a long time (for example, a family reunion), show photographs of the people who will be there and review their names.

• Suggest having trusted friends or adults nearby to provide prompts or facilitate communication.

ADVOCATING

There is no trickier place to advocate for oneself than in the social arena. We'd add that there is possibly no question that is fraught with more concern for parents than "Does my child fit in?" Advocating for themselves is crucially important for kids with slow processing speed because most people don't understand why they act the way they do. For instance, Paul was a bright fourth grader who had ADHD and very slow processing speed. On the bus one morning, the fourth- and fifth-grade boys who were seated near him kept putting their feet out into the aisle so that people would trip. These weren't malicious acts but would rather fall into the category of "thoughtless things that 9- and 10-year-old boys do." Interestingly, no one fell. The boys put their feet out in the aisle but quickly pulled them in right before the person would have tripped. Well, at least until Paul started participating in these high jinx.

It's worth noting that Paul was the very last boy to engage in this behavior. It took him a while to figure out what the "game" was. When he finally started putting his feet into the aisle, most of the other boys had stopped because they realized the bus driver was on to them. Paul was a bit late in understanding all of this, so he didn't stop. More upsetting, when he did put his foot out in the aisle, he didn't pull it back in time, and a sweet first-grade boy tripped and fell. The first-grade boy cried all the way to school, and when he got to school and told the teacher what had happened, guess who got in trouble? Was it the boys who had started the "game"? Were they implicated at all? The answer to both questions is "no."

So what happened to Paul? Well, he was called to the principal's office, where a particularly unempathic principal, Ms. Young, pelted Paul with questions: "Why did you do that? Are you some kind of bully?" Paul sat there absolutely mute. There was no way he could organize his thoughts and respond. Ms. Young thought Paul's silence was belligerence. She assumed he was the instigator and called his mother. Paul's mother felt terrible that this had happened. Tripping kids on the bus didn't sound like Paul at all, and neither did the label of *belligerence*.

When Paul got home, he explained the situation to his mom and started by saying, "Mom, am I going to jail for this?" and "What is juvie hall?" He was pretty traumatized because Ms. Young had started yelling at him, "Do you know where boys who do these things go? Have you heard of juvenile hall? Do you want me to get the police?" Of course, emotionally charged questions like this had only slowed Paul's ability to respond even further. At this point, Paul's mother had two problems on her hands. First, she needed to help Paul understand that what he and the other boys did was wrong. Second, she had to help Ms. Young understand that her reaction to the problem was wrong too. In fact, Paul's mom needed to advocate for Paul in a way that would help Ms. Young understand her son better.

In this case, Paul's mom was advocating for Paul after the fact. It might have been a better idea for her to have made yearly appointments with the principal so that Ms. Young was more aware of his profile. As a result of this incident, Paul's mom made sure to make yearly appointments with the school staff, in addition to the IEP meeting, to discuss Paul's progress, learning style, and appropriate accommodations. But Paul's mom also realized that Paul needed to have been a better advocate for himself, as well as being a better judge of his behavior.

As Paul's story indicates, grade school is not too early to start helping your child become comfortable speaking up for herself in social situations because these skills can often become more difficult to acquire later on, during the self-conscious middle and high school years. As early as kindergarten or first grade, you can guide your child to better self-advocacy by engaging the child in the following ways:

- Encourage your child to express his needs in everyday activities. For example, at a restaurant, rather than reading the menu (or worse, ordering for him because he was too slow to make up his mind), have him read the menu and make his own choices.

- When you go to the store together, have your child ask the sales clerk where her favorite ice cream is located or where the toy section is located. When she's done, give her feedback on her interactions: *Did she speak up so that the clerk could hear her? Did she make eye contact? Did she accurately perceive the information the clerk gave her?*

- Try to anticipate the kinds of situations in which your child will need to advocate for his own needs and role-play those with him. For instance, if it's a new school year and he's starting middle school, help him prepare how to talk to each of his teachers about getting extended time on tests, as is documented in his IEP. Role-play scenarios that may come up at school, such as a pop quiz that he can't finish in time, or not being able to copy his assignment in his notebook before he needs to leave for his next class.

- Encourage your child to be as specific as possible when approaching a teacher. Saying "I can't write down the assignment" isn't as effective as "I have trouble writing things down quickly, and my IEP says that I can get help with this if I can't do it on my own. What's the best way for me to make sure I have the right assignments every day?" Your child may not be able to do this until adolescence, but it is a good skill to learn as early as possible.

- The most important step in teaching self-advocacy is teaching children to understand themselves. Help your child take inventory of her social strengths and weaknesses. Self-analysis can be the most difficult step in the self-advocacy process, and this is especially the case in the emotional-filled social realm.

Obviously, your child's ability to apply the preceding ideas depends on age and maturity.

What If Your Child Is Being Bullied?

We know of no data that would indicate that kids with slow processing speed are bullied more than those without. However, statistics have shown that one out of four kids is bullied and that kids are targeted for bullying based on some type of real or perceived difference, with the most common being different size, different from the majority population, or different ability (that

"What can I do if, like my child, I struggle socially? Who can help?" We've mentioned this issue before—sometimes the apple doesn't fall far from the tree—which means it is not uncommon for parents of children with social difficulties to complain that they have the same problems. They report being shy or just not fitting in, and that they too struggled to make friends. So, in these cases, what is a parent to do? We offer the following suggestions:

- Enlist the help of a socially skilled family member to support your child, such as a "cool uncle" or socially skilled sister-in-law.
- Sign your child up for camp or an afterschool program; alert the leaders of these groups that your child might need some extra help socially.
- Think about enrolling your child in a social skills group for children—that is, a group that is specifically designed to teach your child social skills.
- Inquire whether or not your child could have a peer "mentor" at school, such as an older student or a more socially skilled student, who could help your child socially.

is, the target of the bullying appears to be the kind of child who doesn't seem like she'll stand up for herself). A typical "target" child has something that makes her stand out, like a disability that makes her walk or talk differently. Kids with slow processing speed often fall into that category. In terms of what your child can do, the best advice is to teach your child the following:

- Ignore the bully.
- Don't cry, get angry, or get upset (at least not outwardly), if possible.
- Respond as nonchalantly and firmly as possible to the

bully, by saying things such as "That's not true" or "You're wrong about that."

- Remove yourself from the situation and go to a location where an adult is present.

- You are not the one with the problem. It's the bully who has the problem.

Other, more practical suggestions include teaching your child these tips:

- Always have a friend around when walking to or from school.

- Avoid places where bullying happens, such as unsupervised areas of the school.

- If bullying happens on the school bus, sit near the front of the bus, near the bus driver.

- Don't take expensive things or money to school.

- Label belongings with permanent marker so if they do get stolen (and found), you'll be able to identify them.

As a parent of a child who is bullied, you might find yourself ready to march into your child's school and scream at the child who was mean to your child. Luckily, though, most parents don't do this. It's a good thing, because one of the biggest complaints we hear from kids is that they don't like their parents meddling in their friendships and embarrassing them in front of their teachers or school staff. Instead of getting angry, lend support by doing some of the following:

- Lend a sympathetic ear. Empathize without scaring your child that you're going to jump into action. Sometimes kids just want someone to listen and agree.

- Resist the temptation to solve your child's problems by picking up the phone and calling the alleged bully's mother.

Help your child strategize a way out that feels comfortable for her.

- Brainstorm bully comebacks ahead of time and practice them with your child.

- Give your child the home setting that allows him to act and feel confident. Teach him to hold his head up, stand up straight, and make eye contact.

We do have one important caveat to this advice: If your child is being bullied to the point where he is avoiding school, showing signs of depression or anxiety, or you are worried about his safety, don't be silent. If bullying is more than just a passing concern, we urge you to consult the reference books listed in Resources (pages 185–195) for more information about this important topic.

Finally, parents of kids with slow processing speed frequently ask what they should watch out for with regard to social skills. Since the area of social skills is very much dependent on developmental age, we've broken it down to particular age groups in the checklist on pages 138–140. Feel free to photocopy the form for additional uses, or you can download it from *www.guilford.com/*

PRACTICAL STRATEGIES FOR ACCOMMODATING SOCIAL SKILLS DEFICITS IN CHILDREN WITH SLOW PROCESSING SPEED

Simplify social situations and provide guidance.

- Scaffold and support your child's social interactions with others.
- Provide supports for your child to organize his thoughts and assist in effective communication with peers.
- Assist your child during fast-paced and complex social situations.

braaten3-forms. If you find yourself checking many of the items listed for the child's age, it might be time to address this issue in a more formal way, through therapy, social skills training, or some of the techniques we've outlined in this chapter.

Slow Processing Speed and Friendships: What to Look Out for at Different Ages

3 to 5 years old

- ❑ Slow to join group activities
- ❑ Has trouble getting started on an activity with a friend (for example, seeming lost when a friend comes over to play)
- ❑ Has difficulty remembering and retrieving "social information," such as any details from a playdate or something as simple as a friend's name
- ❑ Has trouble following along during an imaginative scenario with a friend
- ❑ Acts shy, seems quiet, or appears lost in his or her own thoughts
- ❑ Avoids playing with others in fast-paced or busy situations, such as in a crowded waiting room with many children and limited toys
- ❑ Is the "follower" during social times, frequently a step behind and/or simply copying the behaviors of other children
- ❑ Stares blankly at a friend, teacher, or parent
- ❑ Is described by preschool teachers as a "loner" or being less interactive than the other children
- ❑ Has trouble picking up on the rules of social games, such as tag or duck, duck, goose
- ❑ Engages in solitary activity (for example, looking for clovers in the field) versus playing with others
- ❑ Has trouble shifting quickly from one social activity to another (for example, slow to move from the sandbox to a sing-along in circle time)
- ❑ Has trouble responding to his or her name when it is called

(cont.)

Slow Processing Speed and Friendships *(cont.)*

6 to 12 years old

☐ Is chosen last by peers during organized activities (for example, kickball)

☐ Is slow to pick up on social cues (for example, when a friend is getting subtly annoyed)

☐ Has trouble remembering rules to organized games (for example, capture the flag) or missing out on key instructions

☐ Has difficulties telling clear and concise stories to others

☐ Is slow to join group activities

☐ Has trouble independently organizing a playdate

☐ Comes across as stilted or awkward during social interactions

☐ Seems a "beat" behind when laughing at jokes or responding to sarcasm

☐ Complains that certain social situations (for example, indoor playground at McDonald's) are "too loud" or overwhelming

☐ Doesn't notice when friends have arrived or left during busy social situations

☐ Has difficulty independently coming up with ideas of what to play with a friend

☐ Is described by teachers as a "wallflower" or as "not being on the same wavelength as others"

☐ Has trouble remembering to get information needed to set up a playdate, such as a friend's last name or phone number

☐ Has difficulty coming up with what to say during small talk and social chit-chat

☐ "Drifts off" when others are talking quickly or presenting many ideas at once

13 years and older

☐ Has difficulties with group assignments due to slow speed of work completion

☐ Forgets to RSVP to organized parties or events

(cont.)

Slow Processing Speed and Friendships *(cont.)*

- ❑ Forgets dates and times of important social events (for example, school dance)
- ❑ Has trouble picking up on subtle social cues from friends
- ❑ Has difficulties "getting to the point" when telling a story
- ❑ Annoys others by always running late
- ❑ Has problems remembering tickets and passes for important events with friends (for example, concerts)
- ❑ Asks the same questions of his friends multiple times (for example, "What time are we meeting Carrie again?")
- ❑ Has trouble organizing group activities
- ❑ Misreads social cues
- ❑ Has trouble following complex stories told by friends
- ❑ Is slow to respond to text messages and e-mails from friends
- ❑ Misses out on social activities due to slow pace of homework/chore completion
- ❑ Has trouble remembering information about current events and conversation topics
- ❑ "Hangs back" at parties and other fast-paced social situations

The Emotional Costs of Slow Processing Speed

As you've read by now, having slow processing speed can take a toll on a child's academic progress, social relationships, and family dynamics. The cumulative cost of having had difficulties in these far-reaching domains can result in problems in the emotional realm. It's not that problems with slow processing speed directly cause a child to be depressed, but that chronically feeling behind or less skilled (socially or academically) than peers can lead to feelings of depression and anxiety.

We first evaluated 16-year-old Jeffrey when he was 5 years old. At that time he was having difficulty adjusting to the social and behavioral demands of kindergarten. His first evaluation indicated that he was at risk for a learning disability or ADHD, and one significant aspect of his profile indicated problems with processing speed. Subsequent evaluations showed that Jeffrey did meet criteria for ADHD, but the most significant and consistent aspect of his profile was slow processing speed. His classroom performance over the years was inconsistent. When he had an understanding teacher, he performed well and was happy. When he was placed with teachers who didn't understand his learning style and needs, he had a tendency to become mildly depressed and anxious. He had never needed treatment for depression and anxiety, however, because once the school year ended his mood always improved.

This last school year was different. When Jeffrey's mom, Eloise, called us for advice, he had just completed his sophomore year of high school and, unlike in other years, this summer Jeffrey didn't start feeling better. In fact, he was having difficulty getting out of bed in the morning. When his report card came in the mail 2 weeks after school had ended, he had one F, a D+, and the rest were C's. His F was in physics, and although his physics teacher said that he had the ability to be at least a B student in the class, Jeffrey couldn't keep up with the content of the class because he was late almost every morning. Between absences and frequent tardiness, he couldn't keep up. His inability to get to class on time was more than just slowness—he was depressed—and his mother knew she needed to get help, which prompted her call to us.

Jeffrey's case isn't unique. Our research has shown that over one-third of the children in our sample who have slow processing speed also have problems with mood, such as depression, mood swings, and feelings of hopelessness. This is not just the typical moodiness observed in all children at one time or another, but clinically significant mood problems that warrant a diagnosis of depression or mood dysregulation. Additionally, one-third of our sample also met criteria for an anxiety disorder. This research is correlational, meaning that we've shown there is an association between slow processing speed and anxiety and depression, but one doesn't necessarily cause the other. However, it's not a stretch to hypothesize that the effect of struggling to meet the demands of parents, teachers, and friends can cause a child to feel depressed, anxious, and just generally down on himself.

Emotional Problems Frequently Seen in Kids with Slow Processing Speed

LOW SELF-ESTEEM

Self-esteem, or self-worth, is the armor that we wear to protect us from the trials and tribulations of life. Self-esteem fluctuates as kids grow, but it's shaped by our experiences and perceptions. Most children struggle with low self-esteem at one time or another, but when a child has slow processing speed, a "struggle" can become more of a chronic problem.

John was an athletic ninth-grade student who performed better on the football field than in the classroom. He was a puzzle to his parents and teachers because he could remember the plays that he and his team practiced but couldn't remember the material on the Spanish test. His coach thought he had real talent but was forced to bench him on multiple occasions because he was late for practice or on academic probation for failing two classes. This did not have the effect of humbling John; rather, he had a tendency to act *overconfident* at these times, boasting that he was the best on the team but that his "idiot teachers" were "out to get" him. This overconfidence was just a veneer that hid significant problems with self-esteem that were obvious only to his parents, who bore the brunt of his irritability and anger.

In many ways John had internalized his failures. Underneath the bravado he thought of himself as one big problem and suffered from low self-esteem. He coped with these feelings in one of two ways—by acting overconfident or completely demoralized. He'd alternate between saying "That coach doesn't know what he's doing—I'm the best person on that team" and "I can't do anything right. I hate football, and I don't care if I ever play again."

Children and adults with low self-esteem tend to have a low tolerance for frustration and to be easily critical or disappointed in themselves. Like John, they tend to give up easily and sometimes externalize blame for their failures. Most troubling, kids with poor self-esteem tend to see temporary setbacks as permanent and can become chronically pessimistic. Poor self-esteem has been linked to mental health problems, particularly depression.

DEPRESSION

As we indicated earlier, about a third of the children in our sample with slow processing speed also met criteria for a mood disorder, particularly depression. With so many experiences of frustration and failure, some children with slow processing speed might begin to feel hopeless about the future. This was true in the case of Jeffrey. Like Jeffrey, children with slow processing speed and depression may struggle to find motivation and develop a "Why should I care?" kind of attitude. They might be more irritable around the house, become tearful more quickly, or seem overly sensitive. You might notice more physical complaints, such as headaches or stomachaches, or sleep problems, like trouble falling asleep or waking up in the morning.

Depression in children looks different from depression in adults. When you think about depression, you might get a picture in your head of someone who is sad, cries all the time, mopes around the house, and confines herself to her room. But this is not necessarily what depression looks like in children. Children are more likely than adults to express their mood through *behavior*. They may act out toward others (for example, start fights), pick on their siblings, be quick to anger, or not listen to you or follow rules at home.

ANXIETY

Whereas some children experience feelings of depression related to their slow speed, others may develop anxiety. Instead of feeling hopeless, they worry more. They might become overconcerned about their performance, worry about what others think of them, or get easily worked up by little things—especially things having to do with *time*, such as running late or completing a test on time. They may even overcompensate for their slow processing speed with perfectionism. They might stay up for hours, slowly plugging away at their homework; get worked up about upcoming tests; and not turn in projects until they are absolutely perfect.

Take the case of Emma, a 9-year-old girl we saw for an evaluation. Emma was having a hard time getting her work done in class, and her teacher brought up this issue with her parents. Emma's teacher thought she seemed distracted, and in-class work was taking her at least twice as long to finish as her classmates.

On spelling tests and math drills, Emma would "know her stuff" when she practiced with her parents at home but then would forget everything upon testing at school.

Emma started complaining about going to school in the mornings, saying she felt sick. When her parents asked if she was concerned about something, she denied feeling worried, but she said she just "felt bad." She started to have problems falling asleep at night and didn't like to be away from her parents. If her mother happened to be late coming home from work, Emma would sit by the window looking out and think the worst, like that her mother had gotten into a car accident or died. In Emma's situation, slow processing speed was just a piece of the puzzle in what was an underlying anxiety disorder; however, when she received treatment at school and in counseling, this aspect of her profile was an important one to consider. In other words, when therapies were put into place to treat her problems with anxiety, the therapist, tutor, or teacher needed to remember that it might take Emma longer to put those practices into place.

To form a preliminary idea of whether your child might have emotional problems related to slow processing speed, use the checklist on pages 146–147. You can photocopy it to use it for more than one child or download it from *www.guilford.com/braaten3-forms*.

Accepting the Vicious Cycle of Slow Processing Speed and Emotional Difficulties

Remember those three A's of processing speed? Well, acceptance is key, but in the case of emotional difficulties, it can be a tall order. We mentioned above that just because there's an *association* between slow processing speed and emotional difficulties, one does not necessarily cause the other, yet parents constantly wonder "Was there something more I could have done so that she wouldn't have gotten depressed?" Depression and anxiety tend to be areas where many parents think their kids should be able to "snap out of it." For instance, Jeffrey's mom remarked, "I know

The Emotional Costs of Slow Processing Speed: What to Watch Out For

Check off the signs below that you see on a regular basis in your child.

Low Self-Esteem

- ❑ Is overly boastful
- ❑ Shows a pessimistic or "glass half empty" attitude
- ❑ Complains "No one likes me"
- ❑ Frequently compares him- or herself to others
- ❑ Is overly sensitive to even slight criticism
- ❑ Is embarrassed to show assignments and other projects to teachers/ parents
- ❑ Seems too confident
- ❑ Cannot admit wrongdoing
- ❑ Is too hard on him- or herself
- ❑ Makes self-deprecating comments such as "I'm stupid" or "I'm not good at anything"

Depressive Symptoms

- ❑ Has sleep problems or difficulty waking up in the morning
- ❑ Seems hopeless about the future
- ❑ Has changed appetite or eating habits, eating less or more
- ❑ Acts testy and "short-fused"
- ❑ Expresses feelings of sadness
- ❑ Is overly tearful
- ❑ Behaves aggressively and defiantly at home
- ❑ No longer seems interested in activities and events formerly favored
- ❑ Withdraws from friends and family members
- ❑ Complains of difficulties concentrating at school
- ❑ Seems overreactive to little things

(cont.)

The Emotional Costs of Slow Processing Speed *(cont.)*

❑ Has trouble getting motivated and shows extreme procrastination

❑ Complains of stomachaches, headaches, or other aches and pains

❑ Seems slowed down and lethargic

Anxiety Symptoms

❑ Seems overconcerned about abilities and performance

❑ Demonstrates excessive worry, even over small things

❑ Likes things to be predictable and has trouble with change

❑ Seems uncomfortable meeting new people

❑ Has multiple fears

❑ Refuses to go to school

❑ Complains of stomachaches and headaches

❑ Has trouble being away from parents

❑ Worries about death and harm befalling family members

❑ Has trouble speaking up in class

❑ Experiences repetitive and uncontrollable thoughts and behaviors (for example, counting things over and over)

the owner of the bagel shop in town, and she said she'd hire Jeffrey, but he won't even go down there and fill out the paperwork. I know he'd feel better if he were working." She's right. He might feel better once he's working, but right now he's too depressed and feeling too hopeless even to work part-time at a bagel shop.

There are many wonderful books written for parents about depression and anxiety (such as those we recommend in Resources, pages 189–195) that can help you better understand depression and anxiety. It's key for you to know what it is so that you can accept that it's happening in your child—as well as to know what to expect and how best to treat it. If your child is struggling in this area, we recommend getting a thorough evaluation that considers not only cognitive and academic functioning, but emotional functioning as well. You'll want to make sure you have a solid understanding of how your child's slow processing speed is thought to interact with any types of emotional problems that may be occurring.

The relationship between processing speed and emotional difficulties is complicated. Although slow processing speed may give rise to emotional struggles, the reverse is also true: Emotional struggles may give rise to slowed speed. We call this the *vicious cycle* of slow processing speed and emotional difficulties (see diagram below). Children with slow processing speed are at risk for lower self-esteem, depression, and anxiety—and, if these emotional difficulties arise, they slow down children even further. For instance, we know that children with *depression* often have lower motivation and poorer concentration. If motivation and focus are poor, this will further slow an already slow processing speed. The cycle of slow processing speed and *anxiety* is also a vicious one. Slow processing speed may give rise to anxiety, and then anxiety itself can cause problems with quickly processing information.

You are probably familiar with this phenomenon from your

Slow processing speed

Problems in daily life
• Academic troubles
• Family stress
• Peer problems

Psychological consequences
• Hypervigilance
• Perfectionism
• Low motivation
• Depletion of cognitive resources
• Lethargy

Emotional difficulties
• Low self-esteem
• Depression
• Anxiety

own experience. When riddled with worry, it can be hard to concentrate, listen to others, and get work done. High levels of anxiety can cripple performance, even when the task is simple. We see this all the time in our offices. Children with slow processing speed get worried about their performance, especially on the timed tests we give. Then this anxiety hinders their speed even more, slowing them down or, in more extreme cases, leading to complete refusal to take a particular test.

Accommodating Emotional Difficulties in Children with Slow Processing Speed

There are hundreds of treatments for depression and anxiety in children, and most of the effective treatments would be appropriate for children with slow processing speed who also struggle with these issues. If you think your child is significantly depressed or anxious, you should seek treatment. The accommodations discussed here are ones that you can implement on a daily basis and tend to be useful techniques even for kids who aren't struggling with emotional problems.

TONE DOWN EMOTIONAL CONVERSATIONS

Every family argues and gets emotional, and for some kids it's not a problem. For kids with slow processing speed, arguments and emotionality can make life harder than it should be. Some researchers have devoted their entire careers to studying family arguments, such as what families commonly argue about and how they communicate when things get heated. Studies have shown that when family members argue, both volume and rate of speech increase dramatically—as much as two to three times—which should be no shock to anyone who's had a passionate discussion or disagreement with someone. Research also tells us that family arguments are more frequent when a child is struggling with an emotional issue, such as depression or anxiety. Although family arguments are stressful for all involved, they can be especially stressful for a child with slow processing speed. The whole reason the family is even having an argument in the first place may be lost on a child with slow processing speed: The argument may be moving too quickly for this child to follow—he might have missed the whole point of why Mom is so upset with him to begin with.

Then there is the problem of keeping up with the *pace* of an argument or family disagreement. The more people involved in the argument, the harder it is to keep track of the situation. The parents of Tessa, a 10-year-old girl with slow processing speed, often misread her behavior as "quietly defiant." When she would get into trouble at home, her parents would shout, "Tessa, why in the world would you do that? What were you thinking?" Tessa would freeze and struggle to come up with an answer; she was still working on figuring out why her parents were mad in the first place. When she stood there frozen and without an answer, Tessa's parents saw this as defiance; their take was that she was being "fresh" and obstinate.

We helped Tessa's parents understand that because of her slow processing speed (and her anxiety, as it turned out), family arguments and emotion-laden questions were very tough for her to handle. We recommended *slowing down* and *toning down* conversations at home, which we knew was going to be difficult. We suggested that when things felt heated at home, the family members involved take a "cooling off" period before trying to talk about it—and maybe revisit the issue once everyone was more collected, could speak more slowly, and could soften the tone. We hoped this shift would spare Tessa increased anxiety and reduce family stress overall.

HELP FIND AN AREA OF SUCCESS

As we mentioned earlier in this chapter, children with slow processing speed might struggle with low self-esteem in part because they often have a hard time in school. All children need their "one thing"— a skill or talent in which they shine; something at which they are the best. Many children shine in academics, although this is often *not* the case for children with slow processing speed.

These children may therefore need to look outside of academics for sources of success.

Take the case of Callie, a 7-year-old girl with slow processing speed and a reading disability. She was struggling in second grade and received special tutoring three times a week in school. She had to be pulled out of class for this tutoring, which made her feel self-conscious. Her parents were worried about Callie's self-esteem. She was asking a lot of questions, such as "Why do I have to be pulled out of class?" and "Why can't I read like other kids?" Although Callie was not an academic superstar, she had a great imagination and loved dressing up, singing, and putting on shows for her family. Callie's parents decided to enroll her in a children's theater group, and Callie thrived. She was the best singer and actress in her group and received a ton of positive feedback from her group director and from friends and family. Theater became Callie's "thing"—and this successful area helped to thwart any negative blows to her self-esteem from her lack of success at school.

INCREASE THE FREQUENCY OF FUN

For children suffering from the emotional costs of slow processing speed, a large portion of the day may be spent worrying or feeling down. Also, since so much time is spent in school, children with slow processing speed often spend most of their days doing something that is not their strong suit. As an adult, you can think of it as being like having a job for which you have very little skill, worse, a job where you realize that your coworkers are much more efficient than you. You can imagine that this would start to wear on your self-esteem and mood over the years.

In research on child anxiety and depression, studies show that one helpful strategy parents can use at home is called *behavioral activation*. The idea behind behavioral activation is to *increase the frequency of fun and enjoyable activities for your child*. The more time your child is doing something enjoyable—playing basketball, spending time with friends, walking with you to a store to pick up an ice cream—the less time she will spend feeling depressed.

You would want to be careful not to pick activities that involve fast processing speed, of course. For instance, a child with slow processing speed and feelings of low self-esteem might not find it fun to play a fast-paced board game with the whole family.

THINK ABOUT THERAPY—
WITH THE RIGHT THERAPIST

If you checked off some of the emotional symptoms on "The Emotional Costs of Processing Speed" form earlier in this chapter, it might not be a bad idea to think about finding a therapist to talk with your child. Talk therapy is actually one of the most effective treatments for anxiety and depression in kids. Child psychologists, social workers, and school counselors do talk therapy. One of the most common approaches used to treat anxiety and depression is called *cognitive-behavioral therapy* (CBT). A therapist using a CBT approach helps children modify their thoughts and actions to reduce anxiety and improve their mood. CBT therapists help children identify and modify the inaccurate thoughts that trigger depressed and anxious feelings. They also help to improve problem-solving strategies and will work with your child to find better ways to cope with stress.

But who is the right therapist for your child? This is a common question we get from parents—and we understand why, because therapist–child fit or "match" is critical to helping your child get the most of his therapy experience. For children with slow processing speed, think about looking for a therapist who:

- Is calming and relaxed.

- Has a gentle demeanor.

- Does not speak too quickly or too loudly.

- Has experience working with children who have cognitive deficits, such as slow processing speed or executive functioning weaknesses.

- Does not present too many ideas at one time.

- Has patience and allows time for your child to think about responses to questions.

- Is someone your child likes seeing.

- Is easy to understand and has organized thinking.

- Uses multiple ways of presenting information to your child in therapy, such as diagrams, handouts, or multimedia.

Advocating for Children with Slow Processing Speed and Emotional Concerns

At this point in this book, you've realized that you are going to be your child's best advocate, especially when it comes to helping others understand your child's unique qualities. We've mentioned in previous chapters that children with slow processing

---

COULD MEDICATION BE HELPFUL?

The decision to use medications for depression or anxiety is often a hard one for parents. You'll need to think about your values and beliefs concerning the use of medication and ultimately decide whether or not to travel down this path. It is important to gather accurate facts about medication treatments for kids with depression and anxiety. There are many scary stories and misinformation on the Internet. Therefore, a *consultation with a child psychiatrist*, who is a specialist in medication treatments for emotional problems in children, would be a good first step. A child psychiatrist can help answer questions you have about the medications and talk with you and your child about possible side effects. Similar to CBT, antidepressant and antianxiety medications effectively decrease symptoms in about three-quarters of children and adolescents.

speed have trouble advocating for themselves, and the problems with self-advocacy are intensified when there are emotional issues in the picture as well. Inherent in low self-esteem, depression, and anxiety in these children are problems with speaking up for themselves. Children with low-esteem or depression often lack the motivation or confidence to ask for help; children with anxiety are sometimes too afraid to ask. For these reasons your role as an advocate for your child with emotional struggles is that much more important.

Depression and anxiety in children are often misunderstood, so your first step in advocating for your child may simply be to educate people on what depression and anxiety look like in kids. For example, sometimes schools are quick to label a child with a combination of learning struggles and depression as having a *behavior problem*. It may be helpful to remind school personnel that your child isn't *choosing* to behave badly—that there must be *reasons* for his behavior, such as that the work is too challenging or she is feeling ineffective as a student. If your child had a full assessment done at school, the psychologist who did the testing could help articulate the causes of your child's behavior at school. You could also get a private assessment done to help figure out what factors are contributing to your child's behaviors at school.

Another step in advocating for your child might be to get emotional supports in place at school. Just as children with learning disabilities are legally entitled to receive help at school, so are children who struggle with emotional difficulties. If your child has a diagnosed emotional difficulty, such as depression or anxiety, she could qualify for certain types of support at school. These supports have two goals: (1) to *directly* help accommodate and lift your child's emotional symptoms at school and (2) to offset the difficulties *associated* with emotional struggles, such as slow speed of completing tests. Supports a child may qualify for include:

- Access to counseling at school on a weekly basis

- Designating a "safe person" to whom a child can go if feeling anxious or overwhelmed

- Frequent praise for a job well done

- Use of positive reinforcements (for example, rewards) versus negative consequences (for example, being sent to the principal's office) to improve behavior or compliance in the classroom

- Extended time on tests and a reduced homework load

- *Not* putting the child in situations that could lead to public embarrassment, such as having him speak in front of the class

- Increasing feelings of success in the classroom by giving the child "jobs" (for example, feeding the class hamster) that are easily completed and fun

- Homework support at the end of the day to help the child get started on tasks and study for tests

- Frequent parent–teacher communication to ensure that everyone is on the same page

Parents also frequently ask us what they should say to their child about struggles with depression and anxiety: "Should I use the word *anxious* or *depressed*?" "Should I talk about it at all with my son?" "What should I say to my daughter?" "How should I say it?"

It is difficult for us to come up with the perfect script dictating exactly what to say because it will depend partly on your child's age. You wouldn't talk to a 6-year-old about her anxiety in the same way you would talk to a 16-year-old. In talking with younger children about how they are feeling, labeling their feelings can actually be quite helpful. You can use words such as *worry* instead of anxiety or *sad* instead of depressed because most young children are more familiar with these words. For instance, when working with young children in our offices, we sometimes call anxiety the "worry dragon" or the "worry monster" and talk about ways to "tame" these creatures.

When talking with adolescents about emotional issues, it

is generally helpful to be pretty open and honest. Be an active listener without interrupting and get a sense of what your teen thinks is going on and why. You might be surprised at the teen's level of insight. On the other hand, you might also find that your teenager isn't ready to talk at all. The critical accomplishment, however, is that you have *opened the lines of communication*. When you talk with your child about feelings of stress and worry, no matter what the child's age, it is important to offer hope. In addition to empathizing with your child, reassure her that things will get better and that these feelings won't last forever. Remind her that she doesn't have to face these feelings alone and that you will work to get her the right help so life can start looking up.

As we end this chapter, it is important to mention that *not all children with slow processing speed have, or will have, emotional struggles* beyond the typical emotional ups and downs of all children. This chapter is not meant to alarm you into thinking that your child will inevitably develop an emotional disorder because of slow speed. Some children will struggle with these issues, whereas others will not. The key is to raise awareness so that, if you do in fact see some emotional symptoms bubbling to the surface, you will have some basic ways of identifying what is happening, why it's happening, and what to do about it.

PART III

Staying Informed

Pulling It All Together: Formally Assessing Processing Speed

As we've recommended, having your child formally assessed by a professional can often be the key to helping you accept, accommodate, and advocate for your child. But what do these reports really look like, and how do you begin to interpret what they mean? Following an evaluation, a professional should sit down with you and explain how your child did, what the scores mean, and what supports should be in place for your child based on his cognitive and academic profile. However, before you go in for this feedback—and before you even start the testing process—it is helpful to know what the final report might look like.

As we mention in Chapter 2, reports can vary widely across clinicians and settings (for example, school reports look different and assess different areas from hospital reports). Here we present samples of two reports from our office: a hospital-based neuropsychological assessment program. We assess many domains of a child's functioning, such as intelligence, attention, language, memory, academics, emotional functioning, and, of course, processing speed. We present reports from two children: Cody, an 8-year-old boy with ADHD, predominantly inattentive type and slow processing speed, and Lisa, a 17-year-old girl with executive functioning weaknesses, including slow processing speed. (These are realistic reports, but all identifying information, including names, ages, scores, gender, and other identifying details, have been changed to protect the privacy of the children on which they are based.)

Sample Report 1: Cody

NEUROPSYCHOLOGICAL EVALUATION

Name: Cody Sumner
Age: 8 years, 5 months
Grade: Third
Date of Birth: 4/7/2004

Reason for Referral

Cody Sumner was referred for neuropsychological testing by his parents at the suggestion of his teacher. Concerns include (1) slow pace of schoolwork completion, (2) sensory integration issues, and (3) symptoms of anxiety (for example, fears, nervousness). The purpose of this evaluation was to obtain a profile of Cody's strengths and weaknesses, clarify diagnoses, and assist with educational and treatment planning.

Background Information

Cody is an 8-year, 5-month-old boy in the third grade at the Greenfield Academy, a private school. Pregnancy with Cody was generally unremarkable, with the exception of marked morning sickness. Delivery was at full term and uneventful. His birth weight was 7 pounds, 9 ounces. Early developmental milestones (that is, crawling, walking, speaking first words) were achieved within expectations. Medical history is notable for seasonal allergies, frequent ear infections, and intermittent constipation. Cody also is frequently faint and complains of stomachaches. Family history is notable for several members with learning disabilities, as per parent report.

Regarding school performance, Cody is described as a very slow worker, who is sometimes "unfocused." In first and second grades, it was thought that Cody was being overly perfectionistic and anxious, and that this was contributing to his slow pace. However, his slow rate of speech and slow pace of task completion have persisted into third grade and appear to be above and beyond perfectionism alone. He sometimes can get stuck or distracted during academic tasks. His teachers have been concerned about his abilities to keep up with his peers.

Despite this slow pace of task completion, Cody's reading and math skills are reportedly advanced, and he shows excellent memory and problem solving skills. However, speeded/timed drills have posed problems for Cody in the past. His parents report that he shows particular difficulty when tested under any sort of timed condition. In the emotional realm, Cody is described as a "worrier" who is often fearful and anxious in new situations. Socially, Cody sometimes has trouble keeping up with the pace of other children. There is also a history of sensory issues (e.g., oversensitivity to certain textures), which were treated with time-limited course occupational therapy.

Behavioral Observations

Cody was tested on one occasion. He is a boy of average height and weight. He was casually dressed and well groomed for the appointment. Affect was within expectations and appropriate. Rapport was easy to establish, as Cody was kind, polite, and cooperated with all requests from the examiner. The most notable observation was that Cody was markedly slow to complete tasks. At times, he appeared internally distracted and his responses to the examiner's comments, jokes, and instructions were slow. That is, there was often a "beat" between the joking of the examiner and a smile/response from Cody. Results of testing are considered a valid representation of his abilities at this time.

WHAT ARE BEHAVIORAL OBSERVATIONS?

Behavioral observations are the neuropsychologist's impressions of your child's behavior before and during the testing. These observations are a neuropsychologist's own judgments based on experiences working with children. The purpose of the observations is to highlight some important aspects of a child's behavior, such as how quickly she worked, what her mood was like on the day of testing, and how she related to the examiner.

Testing Instruments

Wechsler Intelligence Scale for Children, Fourth Edition (WISC-IV); Wechsler Individual Achievement Test, Third Edition (WIAT-III); Beery–Buktenica Developmental Test of Visual–Motor Integration (VMI); Wide Range Assessment of Memory and Learning, Second Edition (WRAML2); Woodcock–Johnson Tests of Achievement, Third Edition (WJA-III)—selected subtests; Woodcock–Johnson Tests of Cognitive Abilities, Third Edition (WJC-III)—selected subtests; Conners Continuous Performance Test–II (CPT-II); Behavior Assessment System for Children, Second Edition—Self Report (BASC-2); Child Behavior Checklist—Parent Report (CBCL); Behavior Rating Inventory of Executive Function—Parent Report (BRIEF-PR); Child Symptom Inventory–4 (CSI-4); Clinical Interview and Review of Records.

Test Results

General Intellectual Functioning

As a measure of intellectual ability, Cody was given the Wechsler Intelligence Scale for Children, Fourth Edition (WISC-IV). The

WISC-IV includes a measure of general intellectual functioning (Full Scale IQ; [FSIQ]), as well as four factor scores. The FSIQ and factor scores are normed to have a mean of 100 and a standard deviation of 15. A standard deviation indicates how much variation or "spread" from the average exists. Cody's scores are reported in the table below.

WISC-IV	Composite score	Percentile rank	Qualitative description
Verbal Comprehension	110	75th	High Average
Perceptual Reasoning	129	97th	Superior
Working Memory	113	81st	High Average
Processing Speed	88	21st	Low Average
Full Scale IQ	**116**	**86th**	**High Average**

Cody showed variable intellectual skills. His verbal skills (that is, vocabulary and general factual knowledge), perceptual reasoning (that is, perceptual pattern analysis), and working memory (that is, ability to hold information in mind to complete a task) were advanced and fell in the high-average to superior range. Processing speed (that is, rate of information processing), however, was a significant area of weakness.

Cody's individual (age-referenced) subtest scores are shown in the tables below. Scores between 8 and 12 are in the average range (mean = 10; standard deviation = 3).

Verbal Comprehension Subtest Scores

Subtests	Scaled score	Percentile rank	Description
Similarities	12	75th	High Average
Vocabulary	11	63rd	Average
Information	13	84th	High Average

Perceptual Reasoning Subtest Scores Summary

Subtests	Scaled score	Percentile rank	Description
Block Design	14	91st	Superior
Picture Concepts	14	91st	Superior
Matrix Reasoning	16	98th	Very Superior

Working Memory Subtest Scores Summary

Subtests	Scaled score	Percentile rank	Description
Digit Span	13	84th	High Average
Letter–Number Sequencing	12	75th	High Average

Processing Speed Subtest Scores Summary

Subtests	Scaled score	Percentile rank	Description
Coding	7	16th	Low Average
Symbol Search	9	37th	Average

Academic Achievement

Cody was administered the Wechsler Individual Achievement Test, Third Edition (WIAT-III), and the selected fluency subtests of the Woodcock–Johnson Tests of Achievement, Third Edition (WJA-III), to determine his performance in the basic areas of academic achievement: reading, mathematics, and spelling. In the following table detailing Cody's WIAT-III scores, both achieved and predicted standard scores are provided (mean = 100; standard deviation = 15), as well as their corresponding percentile and grade equivalents for the achieved scores.

WIAT-III subtest	Standard score	Predicted score	Percentile	Grade equivalent
Word Reading	120	110	91st	5:9
Pseudoword Decoding	126	110	96th	8:1
Basic Reading Composite	*127*	110	*96th*	—
Numerical Operations	117	110	87th	4:5
Math Problem Solving	117	110	87th	4:5
Mathematics Composite	*117*	110	*87th*	—
Spelling	117	110	87th	4:7

WJA-III	Standard score	Percentile	Grade equivalent
Reading Fluency	75	5th	K:8
Mathematics Fluency	75	5th	K:7

WHAT IS "ACADEMIC FLUENCY"?

You might hear from your child's teacher that her "fluency" is slow. This means that your child's *speed* and *accuracy* of completing reading, math, and writing tasks are *slow*. A child may have slow fluency in just one academic area (for example, slow reading fluency) or across all academic areas. Children with slow academic fluency have problems with speeded math drills, timed reading tests, and writing essays within tight time limits.

Regarding *reading* skills, Cody is performing above aptitude- and grade-based expectations, indicating reading abilities are an area of great strength. Further, Cody shows strong performance in the area of *spelling*. Cody's math skills are also above age- and grade-based expectations. Despite these strengths, however, he showed marked difficulty when asked to read and solve math problems under timed conditions (that is, fluency tasks).

Attention, Executive Functioning, and Information Processing

To assess sustained visual *attention*, Cody was administered the Conners Continuous Performance Test–II (CPT–II). On this task, Cody was asked to sustain attention on a set of computerized visual cues, responding as accurately as possible and resisting the impulse to respond when asked not to. Overall, Cody's performance on the CPT–II better matched the performance of a clinical sample of children with ADHD (versus a nonclinical sample). That is, his performance indicated an 89% chance that a clinically significant attention problem exists. His performance was notable for his marked inattentiveness. Further, he was rated by his mother to show many of the inattentive symptoms of ADHD on a diagnostic checklist (mother: 7/9 symptoms endorsed). These

> **"Is there a specific test to determine whether a child has ADHD?"** Unfortunately, evaluators cannot administer just one magical test that can tell whether or not your child has ADHD. However, there are multiple tests that tell evaluators what your child's attention is like compared to his peers (such as the CPT-II mentioned in this report). Evaluators typically use a combination of parent report, teacher report, behavioral observations during the testing, and standardized tests to evaluate a child's attention. When parents, teachers, and the tests of attention all indicate that this is a problem area, a diagnosis of ADHD might be appropriate.

problems included difficulties sustaining attention, problems following through on instructions, and avoiding tasks requiring sustained mental effort. He was also noted to sometimes lose materials necessary for completing activities and was described as forgetful and easily distracted. Regarding Cody's activity level, his mother did not view him as having symptoms of hyperactivity/impulsivity.

Speed of information processing and abilities to rapidly retrieve information were assessed using selected processing subtests of the Woodcock–Johnson Tests of Cognitive Abilities, Third Edition (WJC-III). Results are shown in the following table (mean = 100, standard deviation = 3).

WJC-III	Standard score	Percentile	Age equivalent
Retrieval Fluency	73	4th	5:8
Decision Speed	75	5th	5:9
Rapid Picture Naming	75	5th	5:10
Cognitive Fluency Composite	**73**	**4th**	**5:9**

Findings suggest that Cody has marked difficulty retrieving information rapidly from his mind, quickly making decisions, and processing information quickly. These findings are consistent with parent reports of slow pace of task completion. Further, a parent questionnaire (that is, the Behavior Rating Inventory of Executive Function [BRIEF]), indicated difficulties *planning ahead and organizing* (89th percentile), *attending to and holding information in his mind to complete a task* (95th percentile), and *initiating tasks* (90th percentile).

Fine Motor Skills

Cody is right-handed. To examine motor skills, Cody was asked to complete the Grooved Pegboard, a test wherein pegs with a key on one side must be rotated and inserted quickly into holes. His performance on this task showed an expected right-hand advantage. Further, fine motor speed and accuracy (that is, dexterity) with his dominant hand was in the low average range (Dominant Hand Standard Score = 89, 23rd percentile). Additionally, performance with his left hand was also slow (Non-Dominant Hand Standard Score = 80, 9th percentile).

Memory

Cody's *verbal memory* was assessed using selected subtests of the Wide Range Assessment of Learning, Second Edition (WRAML-2). He performed in the average range when asked to remember details of two stories that were presented verbally (Story Memory Scaled Score = 13, 84th percentile). Further, 20 minutes later, he was able to recognize many key details of these stories (Story Memory Recognition Scaled Score = 15, 95th percentile). He performed in the very superior range when asked to remember words from a list presented to him aloud (Verbal Learning Scaled Score = 18, >99th percentile) and in the high-average range when asked to repeat simple sentences verbatim (Sentence Memory Scaled Score = 13, 84th percentile). Taken together, verbal memory is an area of strength for Cody.

Emotional Functioning

Cody's mother completed the CBCL, where she noted some mild difficulties with anxiety (for example, worries, shows trouble separating from parents; 93rd percentile). His mother also noted that Cody complains of stomachaches, headaches, constipation, and lightheadedness quite frequently. Further, Cody's score was also elevated on the sluggish cognitive tempo scale (>97th percentile). That is, his mother noted that Cody is sometimes "in a fog," frequently daydreams, is slow to complete tasks, and lacks energy.

Summary

Cody Sumner was referred for neuropsychological testing by his parents at the suggestion of his teacher. Concerns include (1) slow pace of schoolwork completion, (2) sensory integration concerns, and (3) symptoms of anxiety (for example, fears, nervousness). The purpose of this evaluation was to obtain a profile of Cody's strengths and weaknesses, clarify diagnoses, and assist with educational and treatment planning.

Results of testing indicate that Cody has many areas of strength. In particular, verbal skills and language-based academics (that is, reading, spelling) are advanced for his age. Further, he is described as creative, kind, and empathic. Overall, he was a delight to test.

Findings from testing also revealed some key areas of weakness. First, as per parent report, behavioral observations, and results of standardized testing, Cody is slow to complete tasks, inattentive, distractible, and a daydreamer. These difficulties have contributed to slow task completion at school, and he reportedly has trouble keeping up with his peers in class. At this time, Cody's difficulties are best conceptualized as *attention-deficit/hyperactivity disorder (ADHD), predominantly inattentive type.*

Processing speed is a particular area of weakness. Like many children with ADHD, Cody is slow to retrieve information from his mind, inattentive to details, slow to make decisions, and has trouble performing well under time pressure. Further, he has difficulty following through on instructions and completing tasks requiring sustained mental effort and is known to lose materials necessary for completing activities and may be distractible. Cody presents with many of these symptoms, and his difficulties have had a significant impact on his functioning in the classroom and socially. Academically, he falters when tested under time constraints. Socially, he is slow to pick up on cues, misses aspects of conversation, and is often not on the same "wavelength" as his peers.

Cody also presents with symptoms of anxiety and fearful-

WHAT IS ADHD?

ADHD is characterized by problems with inattentiveness, impulse control, overactivity, or some combination of all these difficulties. There are three types of ADHD: (1) *predominantly inattentive type*, in which inattention is a concern and hyperactivity/impulsivity is less of an issue; (2) *predominantly hyperactive type*, in which hyperactivity/impulsivity is a concern but sustaining attention is not a major problem; and (3) *combined type*, in which both inattention and hyperactivity/impulsivity are concerns. ADHD affects boys more often than girls and occurs in about 3–5% of school-age children.

ness that appear beyond what would be expected of his developmental level. He has fears of separation and is overly sensitive to scary stimuli (for example, images from television). It is possible that some of these anxiety symptoms might be manifesting somatically for Cody, most notably as stomachaches, tiredness, and feeling faint.

Recommendations

1. Cody will need individualized support, accommodations, and attention in the classroom setting. The following additions and modifications are recommended to encourage his performance at school:

   A. Develop specific, consistent routines to make Cody more aware of expectations; provide a visual schedule for Cody.

   B. Seat Cody in an area close to the teacher and away from possible distractions (for example, distractions outside the window or in the hallway outside the door).

   C. Gain Cody's attention through often-repeated, recognizable cues such as saying his name before giving verbal instructions.

D. Make sure to have Cody's visual attention when giving instructions. He may need frequent verbal and visual reminders to remember to take home assignments, permission forms, etc. Daily communication between Cody's parents and teacher will be essential.

E. Use multiple instructional modalities. Pairing verbal explanations with visual aids, demonstrations, and hands-on experiments is essential for Cody's success.

F. Break down all instructions into manageable segments and present only one or two at a time. Cody will also need additional time to complete tasks, and assignments/tests may need to be modified accordingly. For instance, if it is expected that completing an in-class assignment will take 30 minutes, Cody's assignment should be modified (for example, reducing number of questions) so that he can complete the same assignment in the allotted time.

G. Break long tasks into multiple short tasks. This is most effective when immediate reinforcement is provided for reaching each subgoal leading to the larger goal.

2. Cody's parents are urged to seek consultation with a pediatric neurologist or child psychiatrist regarding findings from this evaluation. The possibility of medication for Cody's attention problems should be discussed with this professional.

3. The following recommendations are suggested to help Cody at home:

A. Allow extra time to do everything. Time constraints and "rushing" may overwhelm and immobilize Cody.

B. Break tasks into manageable components and wait until he has completed one component before giving him further instructions (for example, instead of saying "Clean your room," say, "Put your books on the shelf" and "Put your dirty clothes in the hamper").

C. Provide a consistent schedule. Try to have mealtime, bedtime, etc., occur at the same time and in the same order every day. Inform Cody of any deviations from the routine ahead of time and explain the reason for the change. When traveling away from home, make the new environment as comfortable and familiar as possible.

D. Provide a backup schedule. Help Cody understand that plans are tentative. Say, for example, "We are going to the beach Saturday, unless it rains. If it rains, we will go to the movies."

E. Use a calm voice. Children with attention concerns and anxiety often become worried in response to communication with a high emotional content. Try not to sound intense, passionate, or stressed. Also, try not to raise your voice or yell, as this could be very frightening to Cody. Strive to be logical and sequential.

4. Cody's free time is important to him. Set aside time at the end of the day for Cody to relax and pursue personal interests. Cody should also be encouraged to become involved in activi-

---

"How often should I have my child tested?" The answer here really depends on your child's age, the severity of her difficulties, and the types of problems she may be experiencing. Generally, the younger the child and the more severe the difficulties, the more frequent the evaluations tend to be. A teen who is needing some extra time for tests in an academically rigorous high school may never need another evaluation after 10th grade, whereas a 6-year-old with significant processing speed deficits, ADHD, and an emerging learning disability may need yearly evaluations for the first few years of elementary school. The best advice is to ask the evaluator what he recommends—and be sure to do it. We frequently see parents who regret not following up with recommendations for further assessments.

ties and school-related functions to promote positive relationships.

5. Encourage Cody in areas in which he succeeds. Every child
   needs an area in which to shine. This is particularly important for children with school difficulties, as they often encoun-
   ter frustration in school, which appears to sometimes be the
   case for Cody. His emotional functioning should be monitored
   closely, especially given that children with attention problems
   and early anxiety are at risk of developing a more significant
   emotional issue later on in development. If these problems
   escalate over the course of the year or beyond, his parents
   should seek consultation with a child psychologist.

6. Follow-up testing in approximately 2–3 years is suggested.
   Reevaluations can be used to update interventions based on
   the academic demands he will be facing at that time. This
   is especially important for Cody, as changes in academic
   demands may create a very different symptom presentation.

It was a pleasure to meet with Cody and his family. Cody is a
personable young man, who was a delight to evaluate. Please feel
free to contact us should any questions arise.

Ellen Braaten, PhD
Licensed Psychologist

Brian Willoughby, PhD
Licensed Psychologist

Sample Report 2: Lisa

NEUROPSYCHOLOGICAL EVALUATION

Name: Lisa Clemens
Age: 17 years, 1 month
Grade: Eleventh
Date of Birth: 05/19/1996

Reason for Referral

Lisa was referred for neuropsychological testing by her parents, at the suggestion of her pediatrician, due to variable academic performance last year. Despite being described as a very bright young woman, her average grades fell in the C–D range. The purpose of this evaluation was to clarify the reasons for Lisa's variable academic performance, investigate academic strengths and weaknesses, and assist with educational and treatment planning.

Background Information

Identifying Information

Lisa is a 17-year-old young woman entering 11th grade at a private school in Massachusetts. She lives with her parents, Jackie and

> **"My child never had problems in elementary and middle school. Why is she struggling in high school?"** We frequently see teenagers who sailed through elementary and middle school only to struggle once they hit high school. This may be the case because the demands of high school quickly increase, especially with regard to executive functioning demands (for example, organization, planning ahead, managing multiple subjects at once). Difficulties emerge only in high school because a teen can't handle the increased load of ninth grade (or subsequent grades) on her own.

Michael, and brother (age 4). Her mother completed college and works as a paralegal. Her father completed high school and works as an automotive repairman. English is the only language spoken at home. Lisa's mother served as the primary informant for the background information.

Developmental and Medical Histories

Pregnancy with Lisa was uncomplicated. Delivery was at term. Perinatal history is unremarkable. Developmental milestones, such as turning over, sitting alone, walking, and speaking first words, were achieved within normal limits. Medical history is significant for a mild head injury at age 3 (falling off a swing), although follow-up at a hospital was unremarkable. Asthma and mild hand tremor are also notable. Family medical and psychiatric histories were notable for attention difficulties in a paternal uncle.

Academic History

Academically, Lisa was described by her parents as a bright young woman, who achieved solid grades throughout elementary and middle school. However, despite adequate academic performance, her mother noted that Lisa tended to be disorganized, forgetful, slow to complete tasks, and needed redirection and support for homework completion. During her freshman and sophomore years, she reportedly did well, then her grades faltered. This year, her junior year, she was initially achieving grades in the B range, although her grades slipped as she missed assignments, procrastinated, showed up late to classes, and reportedly lacked initiative.

Social–Emotional History

Lisa is described as a friendly, likable, and even-tempered young woman, with many friends and close connections with family members. There is no reported history of depression, anxiety, aggression, or disruptive behavior concerns. She plays field hockey and basketball at school. She is also involved in dance. As per Lisa, she would like to be a dentist when she is older.

Behavioral Observations

Lisa was tested on one occasion. She is a young woman of average height and weight, who appeared her chronological age. She was casually dressed in a T-shirt, jeans, and sneakers for the testing session and was well groomed. Lisa was alert and cooperative during the examination. Eye contact and reciprocal social smiling were within expectations. She made jokes, laughed with the examiner, and rapport was easily established. Vocabulary and grammar were at a level appropriate for a young woman her age. Attention was generally within expectations, although it was not uncommon for her to need directions repeated. Further, she was very slow to complete tasks. Even when under a time pressure, Lisa worked at an even, slow pace. At times during the clinical interview, Lisa was somewhat guarded and did not elaborate on answers to questions posed by the examiner. She tended to put forth her best effort during the examination and persisted on difficult tasks. Thus, the results of this evaluation are considered a valid representation of Lisa's abilities at this time.

Testing Instruments

Wechsler Adult Intelligence Scale, Fourth Edition (WAIS-IV); Wechsler Individual Achievement Test, Third Edition (WIAT-III); Woodcock–Johnson Tests of Achievement, Third Edition (WJA-III), Fluency subtests; Beery–Buktenica Developmental Test of Visual–Motor Integration (VMI); California Verbal Learning Test, Second Edition (CVLT-II); Delis–Kaplan Executive Function System (DKEFS)—selected subtests; Personality Assessment Inventory—Adolescent (PAI-A); Behavior Assessment System for Children, Second Edition—Parent Report (BASC-2); Behavior Rating Inventory of Executive Function—Parent Report (BRIEF-PR); Behavior Rating Inventory of Executive Function—Self-Report (BRIEF-SR); Child Symptom Inventory–4 Parent Report

(CSI-4); Developmental History Form; Clinical Interview (Lisa/ Mother).

Test Results

General Intellectual Functioning

As a measure of intellectual ability, Lisa was administered the Wechsler Adult Intelligence Scale, Fourth Edition (WAIS-IV). It includes two measures of general intellectual functioning (Full Scale IQ [FSIQ] and General Ability Index [GAI]), as well as four factor scores. The FSIQ and factor scores are normed to have a mean of 100 and a standard deviation of 15. Her scores are reported in the following table.

Scale	Composite score	Percentile rank	Qualitative description
Verbal Comprehension	112	79th	High Average
Perceptual Reasoning	109	73rd	Average
Working Memory	98	45th	Average
Processing Speed	87	19th	Low Average
Full Scale IQ	**104**	**61st**	**Average**
General Ability Index	**109**	**73rd**	**Average**

Overall, Lisa's intellectual abilities fall in the *average to high average* range. However, her FSIQ may not be the best descriptor of her intellectual abilities, given the variability among factor scores. In particular, Lisa's verbal comprehension (that is, general knowledge and vocabulary), perceptual reasoning (that is, perceptual pattern analysis), and working memory (that is, ability to hold information in mind to complete a task) were significantly better than her processing speed (that is, rate of information processing). In fact, 81% of Lisa's peers process information faster than she does. This finding is consistent with behavioral observations, which revealed a very slow rate of task completion. Further, given that Lisa's processing speed served to pull down her FSIQ, it is more appropriate to use the General Ability Index (GAI; a composite of verbal comprehension and perceptual reasoning) as the best indicator of her intellect.

Lisa's individual (age-referenced) subtest scores are shown in the following table. Scores between 8 and 12 are in the average range (mean = 10; standard deviation = 3).

Verbal Comprehension Subtest Scores Summary

Subtests	Scaled score	Percentile rank
Similarities	11	63rd
Vocabulary	13	84th
Comprehension	11	63rd

Perceptual Reasoning Subtest Scores Summary

Subtests	Scaled score	Percentile rank
Block Design	13	84th
Visual Puzzles	11	63rd
Matrix Reasoning	10	50th

Working Memory Subtest Scores Summary

Subtests	Scaled score	Percentile rank
Arithmetic	10	50th
Digit Span*	9	37th

*Digits Forward = 12, Digits Backwards = 7, Sequencing = 9.

Processing Speed Subtest Scores Summary

Subtests	Scaled score	Percentile rank
Coding	8	25th
Symbol Search	7	16th

Achievement Testing

Lisa was administered the selected subtests of the Wechsler Individual Achievement Test, Third Edition (WIAT-III) and Woodcock–Johnson Tests of Achievement (WJA-III) to determine her performance in the basic areas of academic achievement: reading, mathematics, spelling, and writing. In the table detailing Lisa's WIAT-III scores, both achieved and predicted standard scores are provided (mean = 100; standard deviation = 15), as well as their corresponding percentile and grade equivalents for the achieved scores.

WIAT-III subtest	Standard score	Predicted score	Percentile	Grade equivalent
Word Reading	107	96	68th	>12:9
Reading Comprehension	95	96	37th	6:1
Pseudoword Decoding	95	97	37th	8:9
Numerical Operations	91	96	27th	8:4
Spelling	110	96	75th	11:8
Essay Composition	107	96	68th	—

WJA-III subtest	Standard score	Percentile	Grade equivalent
Reading Fluency	84	14th	6:2
Math Fluency	84	14th	6:2

Lisa's word reading, word decoding, computational math, compositional writing, and spelling skills are adequate and generally commensurate with aptitude- and grade-based expectations.

She shows a relative weakness in the area of reading comprehension, in part due to lack of focus on detail when reading passages. Lisa showed the greatest weakness when asked to read and solve math problems under timed conditions. That is, her reading and math fluency fell to the level of a sixth grader. This is not surprising given Lisa's slow processing speed.

Visual Construction Skills

Lisa was administered the Beery–Buktenica Developmental Test of Visual–Motor Integration (VMI), which assesses an individual's visual–motor development, perceptual discrimination ability, and skill at integrating the perceptual and motor processes. This test consists of 24 geometrical forms that are copied in a developmental sequence, from simple to more complex. Lisa was required to copy the figures from examples using a pencil and paper. On the VMI, Lisa's visual–motor abilities tested in the *average* range (Standard Score = 96, 39th percentile).

Memory

To assess memory skills, Lisa was administered the California Verbal Learning Test, Second Edition (CVLT-II). On the CVLT-II, Lisa was read a list of 15 words over five trials. She showed marked difficulty initially encoding an adequate number of words (4/15) and had trouble learning new words over subsequent trials (5, 5, 9). By the fifth and final trial, she had learned 8/15 words, which was below expectations. After presentation of a distracter list and a short delay, she was able to remember only 6/15 words. Even with cueing (for example, reminders about the types of words), she had trouble remembering more words (5/15). Overall, Lisa's performance on the CVLT-II indicates problems encoding verbally based information (that is, taking verbal information "into" memory). These problems are not uncommon among individuals with attention and executive functioning issues. She did much better when asked to remember and draw the Rey Complex Figure (described above) from memory. Therefore, visual memory appears intact.

Attention and Executive Functioning

Lisa's mother reported on her attention and activity level. On the Behavior Assessment System for Children, Second Edition (BASC-2), a standardized instrument that requires parents to evaluate their child's behavior, Lisa was viewed as having mildly elevated levels of inattention (Parent-Reported Inattention = 84th percentile). Further, on a checklist of ADHD symptoms, she was noted to sometimes demonstrate the following: failure to give close attention to details, problems following through on instructions, trouble organizing tasks and keeping track of materials. She was also noted to sometimes be forgetful, easily distracted, careless in her work, and avoidant of tasks requiring sustained mental effort. These problems did not reach the threshold for a clinical diagnosis of ADHD, although they clearly indicate mild attention-related difficulties. With regard to Lisa's activity level, her mother did not view her as hyperactive or impulsive on the BASC-2 or ADHD symptoms checklist.

Lisa's executive functioning (for example, set shifting, organization, initiative) was assessed using standardized tests and parent report. She was administered selected subtests of the Delis–Kaplan Executive Function System (DKEFS). Results are shown in the following table (scaled score mean = 10, standard deviation = 3).

DKEFS subtest	Scaled score	Percentile	Classification
Trails: Motor Speed	4	2nd	Borderline
Trails: Number–Letter Switching	8	25th	Average
Verbal Fluency: Total Correct	5	5th	Borderline
Verbal Fluency: Switching Accuracy	4	2nd	Borderline

On the DKEFS, mild difficulties with executive functioning were revealed. On tasks that required Lisa to quickly shift sets (that is, switch quickly and accurately from one line of thinking to another), she showed difficulty. Further, when asked to switch back and forth between naming fruits and pieces of furniture, she lost track and began naming types of vegetables instead of fruits. She also showed difficulty on a simple test of motor speed.

Lisa's executive functioning was further evaluated with parent and self-report rating scales. On the parent version of the Behavior Rating Inventory of Executive Function (BRIEF-PR), Lisa's mother expressed concerns about her abilities to *attend and hold information in mind to complete a task* (Parent-Reported Working Memory = 97th percentile) and *plan ahead and organize* (Parent-Reported Plan/Organize = 92nd percentile). On the self-report version of this scale, Lisa also noted mild problems with planning and organizing (Plan/Organize = 97th percentile) and task completion (for example, completing homework, Task Completion = 70th percentile). Lisa noted that she doesn't think ahead about possible problems, sometimes begins projects without the correct materials, forgets to hand in her homework even when it is completed, has many unfinished projects, and is slow to complete her work.

Emotional Functioning

Lisa's emotional functioning was evaluated using the Personality Assessment Inventory, Adolescent Version (PAI-A), a self-report questionnaire. Results of the PAI-A did not reveal any evidence of clinical psychopathology. That is, there were no significant problems with the following: antisocial behavior, empathy, suspiciousness or hostility, moodiness, impulsivity, unhappiness or depression, unusually elevated mood, anxiety, health or physical functioning, or alcohol/drug abuse or dependence. Her self-concept appears to involve a generally stable and positive self-evaluation. During the clinical interview, Lisa did note that she had some difficulty adjusting during her first year of high school. Further, she indicated variability in her grades, although she had difficulty identifying the specific reasons for her variable academic performance.

HOW IS EMOTIONAL FUNCTIONING ASSESSED IN ADOLESCENTS?

Emotional functioning can be assessed in a variety of ways. In every evaluation, the evaluator should ask questions of you and your child regarding the child's emotional functioning. Through your answers to these questions, the evaluator determines whether there is a more serious emotional problem that needs to be assessed. If so, the evaluator will use questionnaires and projective tests, such as the Rorschach and the Thematic Apperception Test (TAT). These last two tests require adolescents to describe what they see in an inkblot (Rorschach) and to tell a story about a picture (TAT). Their responses to these types of tests give us ideas about their underlying motives, feelings, and drives. Personality and behavior questionnaires are used in conjunction with projective testing to obtain a comprehensive picture of their psychological, behavioral, and emotional functioning. It can also provide insight into the types of treatments that would be most helpful.

To further evaluate Lisa's emotional functioning, her mother completed the BASC-2 Parent Report. Lisa's mother did not endorse any at-risk or clinically significant problems on this questionnaire. Further, on the Child Symptom Inventory–4 (CSI-4), a diagnostic checklist of possible psychiatric disorders, her mother did not view Lisa as meeting criteria for any specific psychiatric disorders.

Summary

Lisa Clemens is a 17-year-old young woman who was referred for testing by her parents, at the suggestion of her pediatrician, due to variable academic performance. Despite being described as a bright young woman, she earned very poor grades this past year. The purpose of this evaluation was to clarify the reasons for Lisa's variable academic performance, investigate academic strengths and weaknesses, and assist with educational and treatment planning.

Findings from this evaluation reveal that Lisa is a charming, personable, and engaging young woman. She is social, polite, and shows a good sense of humor. Despite these strengths, results of testing indicate a few key areas of weakness that are likely contributing to her current academic struggles. First, results of testing indicate that Lisa has *slow processing speed and executive functioning weaknesses*. That is, she has trouble completing work quickly, planning ahead, organizing, initiating, seeing the big picture, and shifting rapidly from one line of thinking to another. From a neurological perspective, these are all frontal-lobe functions and, in a school setting, manifest as problems planning ahead for long-term projects, remembering to hand in homework, completing class assignments, working well under time pressure, managing time effectively, attending for long periods of time, and working at the same pace as other students. Although Lisa may start off a school year well (likely due to the novelty and slow pace of the first few months), she quickly becomes overwhelmed with her workload and her academic performance falters.

Second, Lisa also presents with mild problems *attending to and "taking in" information*, which makes it difficult for her to remember information that is verbally presented. That is, in comparison to her peers, she has more trouble taking in information and storing the information in a meaningful way so it can be retrieved from memory at a later time. These memory difficulties appear to be related to her executive functioning weaknesses, because not having a system or organizing strategy for remembering information (for example, chunking information by category) can lead to memory problems. This combination of executive functioning, attention, and encoding difficulties is currently contributing to Lisa's suboptimal academic performance, as per testing. Although these problems are common among children and adolescents with attention-deficit/hyperactivity disorder (ADHD), Lisa's symptoms do not reach a level of clinical significance that would qualify her for the disorder at this time. However, it is of note that many of the accommodations and treatments for adolescents with ADD/ADHD may be useful in Lisa's case.

Regarding psychological health, Lisa appears free of any mood, anxiety, or behavioral disturbance at this time. Her self-concept involves a positive self-evaluation. Further, she is a confident and optimistic young woman, who is resilient and adaptive in the face of stressors. As per testing, there is not a clear emotional or psychological issue that would explain her current academic struggles.

Overall, Lisa is a kind, confident, and extraverted young woman with a family that truly cares for her. Based on the results of this evaluation, recommendations follow:

Recommendations

1. Lisa will need accommodations and supports in her current placement to address her executive functioning and memory concerns. To enhance Lisa's general academic performance, the following should be implemented:

   A. Give Lisa additional time to complete homework, assignments, and tests. It is important that she not be penalized for slowness. Further, she would benefit from a reduced homework load and extended time for testing. She also qualifies for 50% extended time testing on standardized tests, such as the SATs.

   B. Seat Lisa near the site of instruction (that is, front of the class).

   C. Instruct Lisa to take frequent breaks if needed.

   D. Give frequent feedback.

   E. Give brief, concise directions.

   F. Give one-on-one check-in time.

G. Provide review and study sheets with key concepts prior to the test.

H. Reduce sources of distraction in the classroom.

I. Remind Lisa to turn in homework or take home materials that are necessary for the completion of homework.

J. Break up long-term assignments into several steps, with specific due dates for each step.

2. Because Lisa has difficulty in the area of executive functions, a tutor would be useful to help teach her organizational, planning, time management, and study skills as well as self-monitoring techniques. If school personnel cannot provide this weekly service, her parents may want to consider hiring a private executive tutor for Lisa. A tutor may also be able to provide extra support and compensatory strategies in the area of reading comprehension, such as reading the questions ahead of time, highlighting key ideas, and making predictions/inferences based on the text.

3. Lisa's free time is important to her. Set aside time at the end of the day for her to relax and pursue personal interests. She should continue to be encouraged to become involved in activities and school-related functions to promote positive relationships.

4. Lisa would benefit from the assistance of technology to facilitate her executive functioning and memory difficulties, such as a watch or phone with a reminder function.

5. Follow-up testing in approximately 2–3 years to monitor Lisa's progress and evaluate the success of recommended interventions is suggested.

It was a pleasure to meet with Lisa and her family. Lisa is a charming and personable young woman, who was a delight to evaluate.

Brian Willoughby, PhD
Licensed Psychologist

Ellen Braaten, PhD
Licensed Psychologist

*   *   *

These sample reports give you a sense of what you might expect if you have your child evaluated by a professional. The recommendations in these reports are key, as the evaluator will tailor the recommendations specifically to your child—and following these recommendations can lead to great improvements! These reports will not only help you better understand your child's strengths and weaknesses, but also help teachers and any other professionals working with your child.

Resources

The following is a listing of additional books, organizations, and websites that might be of interest to parents and professionals supporting children with slow processing speed.

BOOKS FOR PARENTS

These books tackle a range of topics relevant to parents who have children with slow processing speed. Because these children often struggle with attention and other executive functioning issues, many of the books mentioned here cover these topics. ADHD is a common problem among children with slow processing speed, so we mention several books specifically written to help parents understand this diagnosis, as well as treatments for ADHD. Other books listed here are relevant to *testing* for slow processing speed, such as better understanding the neuropsychological assessment process, and *accessing school supports* for children with disabilities.

Barkley, R. (2013). *Taking charge of ADHD: The complete, authoritative guide for parents* (3rd ed.). New York: Guilford Press.

Braaten, E. (2011). *How to find mental health care for your child*. Washington, DC: American Psychological Association.

Braaten, E., & Felopulos, G. (2004). *Straight talk about psychological testing for kids*. New York: Guilford Press.

Byrnes, J. (2001). *Minds, brains, and learning*. New York: Guilford Press.

Coloroso, B. (2008). *The bully, the bullied, and the bystander: From preschool* to high school—how parents and teachers can help break the cycle. New York: Harper Collins.

Cooper-Kahn, J., & Dietzel, L. C. (2008). *Late, lost, and unprepared: A parent's guide to helping children with executive functioning.* Bethesda, MD: Woodbine House.

Cox, A. J. (2007). *No mind left behind: Understanding and fostering executive control—the eight essential brain skills every child needs to thrive.* New York: Penguin.

Dawson, P., & Guare, R. (2009). *Smart but scattered: The revolutionary executive skills approach to helping kids reach their potential.* New York: Guilford Press.

Dawson, P., & Guare, R. (2010). *Executive skills in children and adolescents: A practical guide to assessment and intervention* (2nd ed.). New York: Guilford Press.

Dornbush, M., & Pruitt, S. (2009). *Tigers, too: Executive functions/speed of processing/memory—impact on academic, behavioral, and social functioning of students with ADHD, Tourette syndrome, and OCD.* Marietta, GA: Parkaire Press.

Freedman, J. (2002). *Easing the teasing: Helping your child cope with name-calling, ridicule, and verbal bullying.* New York: Contemporary Books.

Guare, R., Dawson, P., & Guare, C. (2012). *Smart but scattered teens: The "executive skills" program for helping teens reach their potential.* New York: Guilford Press.

Hallowell, E., & Ratey, J. (2011). *Driven to distraction: Recognizing and coping with attention deficit disorder from childhood through adulthood* (rev. ed.). New York: Pantheon Books.

Levine, M. (2004). *The myth of laziness: America's top learning expert shows how kids and parents can become more productive.* New York: Simon & Schuster.

Nigg, J. (2006). *What causes ADHD?: Understanding what goes wrong and why.* New York: Guilford Press.

Smith Myles, B., & Southwick, J. (2005). *Asperger syndrome and difficult moments: Practical solutions for tantrums, range, and meltdowns* (2nd ed.). Mission, KS: Autism Asperger Publishing.

Weinfeld, R., & Davis, M. (2008). *Special needs advocacy resource book: What you can do now to advocate for your exceptional child's education.* Waco, TX: Prufrock Press.

Wilens, T. E. (2008). *Straight talk about psychiatric medications for kids* (3rd ed.). New York: Guilford Press.

Wilmshurst, L., & Brue, A. W. (2005). *A parent's guide to special education: Insider advice on how to navigate the system and help your child succeed* (2nd ed.). San Francisco: Jossey-Bass.

BOOKS FOR TEACHERS AND OTHER PROFESSIONALS

We recommend the following books for teachers and other professionals, such as counselors, social workers, or tutors of children with slow processing speed. These books cover a range of topics, such as effective teaching strategies for children with slow processing speed, learning struggles, and other executive functioning weaknesses. Many of these books outline practical suggestions for helping children with different learning profiles succeed in the classroom environment.

Campbell, B. (2008). *Handbook of differentiated instruction using the multiple intelligences: Lesson plans and more.* Boston: Pearson Allyn & Bacon.

Cooper-Kahn, J., & Foster, M. (2013). *Boosting executive skills in the classroom: A practical guide for educators.* San Francisco: Jossey-Bass.

DeRuvo, S. (2009). *Strategies for teaching adolescents with ADHD: Effective classroom techniques across the content areas.* Hoboken, NJ: Jossey-Bass.

Goldstein, S., & Brooks, R. B. (2007). *Understanding and managing children's classroom behavior: Creating sustainable, resilient classrooms* (Vol. 207). New York: John Wiley & Sons.

McCloskey, G., Perkins, A., & Van Divner, B. (2008). *Assessment and intervention for executive function difficulties.* New York: Routledge.

Meltzer, L. (2007). *Executive function in education: From theory to practice.* New York: Guilford Press.

Meltzer, L. (2010). *Promoting executive function in the classroom.* New York: Guilford Press.

Pfiffner, L. J. (2011). *All about ADHD: The complete practical guide for classroom teachers* (2nd ed.). New York: Scholastic.

Reid, G., & Johnson, J. (2011). *Teacher's guide to ADHD.* New York: Guilford Press.

Smith Myles, B., Adreon, D., & Gitlitz, D. (2006). *Simple strategies that work!: Helpful hints for all educators of students with Asperger syndrome, high-functioning autism, and related disorders.* Mission, KS: Autism Asperger Publishing.

BOOKS FOR KIDS

The following are books that may be helpful for children with slow processing speed. They are "child friendly" books; children can read them alone or with a parent. These books target topics including learning disabilities, attention and executive functioning problems, and simply what it is like to feel "different" from others.

Cook, J. (2011). *The worst day of my life ever!* Boys Town, NE: Boys Town Press.

Esham, B. (2008). *The last to finish: A story about the smartest boy in math class.* Ocean City, MD: Mainstream Connections.

Esham, B. (2013). *Free association: Where my mind goes during science class.* Ocean City, MD: Mainstream Connections.

Gehret, J. (2009). *The don't give up kid and learning disabilities.* Fairport, NY: Verbal Images Press.

LeSieg, T., & Tobey, B. (1993). *I wish that I had duck feet.* New York: Random House.

Levine, M. (1993). *All kinds of minds: A young student's book about learning abilities and learning disorders.* Cambridge, MA: Educators Publishing.

Parr, T. (2009). *It's okay to be different.* New York: Little, Brown.

Pollack, P. (2009). *I can't sit still!: Living with ADHD.* Hauppauge, NY: Barron's Educational Series.

Zobel Nolan, A. (2009). *What I like about me!* New York: Reader's Digest.

WEBSITES

www.learningstore.org

The Learning Store; lists educational products for purchase, designed to help accommodate and assist with learning difficulties and processing issues.

www.chadd.org

Children and Adults with Attention-Deficit/Hyperactivity Disorder; provides information about ADHD, including public policy, legal rights, answers to common questions, and current research in the area.

www.fape.org

Families and Advocates Partnership for Education (FAPE); a partnership aiming to improve the educational outcomes for children with disabilities; links families, advocates, and self-advocates to information about the Individuals with Disabilities Education Act (IDEA).

http://life.familyeducation.com

Provides parenting tips for children of all ages, including topics such as helping your child stay organized and behavior management at home.

www.ncld.org

The National Center for Learning Disabilities; provides descriptions of learning disabilities and processing deficits and how to seek help for these difficulties.

www.disabilityrights.org

The Council for Disability Rights; provides information regarding the rights of people with disabilities, including learning/educational disabilities, and how to advocate for services and supports.

www.smartkidswithld.org

Smart Kids with LD; nonprofit organization dedicated to empowering the parents of children with learning disabilities and ADHD.

www.parentcenterhub.org

The Center for Parent Information and Resources; features research-based information on special education and related topics for parents and professionals; includes a wide selection of news, publication, and resources, as well as a directory of the nation's Parent Centers.

www.learningworksforkids.com

LearningWorks for Kids; provides information regarding executive function skills, specifically offering a detailed explanation of organization and time management skills and technologies to help improve these skills.

www.wrightslaw.com

Wright's Law; provides information about special education law, education law, and advocacy for children with disabilities.

www.ldac-acta.ca

Learning Disability Association of Canada; provides information and resources to help parents of children with learning disabilities in Canada.

http://australia.angloinfo.com/family/schooling-education/special-needs

Special Needs Education in Australia; outlines the kinds of school services available for children with special learning needs in Australia.

www.gov.uk/children-with-special-educational-needs/overview

Children with Special Education Needs; website dedicated to helping understand special education in the United Kingdom.

INTERESTING RESEARCH ON PROCESSING SPEED

Calhoun, S. L., & Mayes, S. D. (2005). Processing speed in children with clinical disorders. *Psychology in the Schools, 42*(4), 333–343.

Gontkovsky, S. T., & Beatty, W. W. (2006). Practical methods for the clinical assessment of information processing speed. *International Journal of Neuroscience, 116*(11), 1317–1325.

Goth-Owens, T. L., Martinez-Torteya, C., Martel, M. M., & Nigg, J. T. (2010). Processing speed weakness in children and adolescents with non-hyperactive but inattentive ADHD (ADD). *Child Neuropsychology, 16*(6), 577–591.

Kail, R. V. (1992). Processing speed, speech rate, and memory. *Developmental Psychology, 28*(5), 899–904.

Kail, R. V., & Ferrer, E. (2007). Processing speed in childhood and adolescence: Longitudinal models for examining developmental change. *Child Development, 78*(6), 1760–1770.

Mayes, S. D., & Calhoun, S. L. (2007). Learning, attention, writing, and processing speed in typical children and children with ADHD, autism, anxiety, depression, and oppositional-defiant disorder. *Child Neuropsychology, 13*(6), 469–493.

Miller, L. T., & Vernon, P. A. (1997). Developmental changes in speed of information processing in young children. *Developmental Psychology, 33*(3), 549–554.

Nettelbeck, T., & Burns, N. R. (2010). Processing speed, working memory, and reasoning ability from childhood to old age. *Personality and Individual Differences, 48*(4), 379–384.

Shanahan, M. A., Pennington, B. F., Yerys, B. E., Scott, A., Boada, R., Willcutt, E. G., et al. (2006). Processing speed deficits in attention deficit/hyperactivity disorder and reading disability. *Journal of Abnormal Child Psychology, 34*(5), 585–602.

Tripp, G., & Wickens, J. R. (2009). Neurobiology of ADHD. *Neuropharmacology, 57*(7–8), 579–589.

Weiler, M. D., Bernstein, J. H., Bellinger, D. C., & Waber, D. P. (2000). Processing speed in children with attention deficit/hyperactivity disorder, inattentive type. *Child Neuropsychology, 6*(3), 218–234.

Index

About the Authors

Ellen Braaten, PhD, is Director of the Learning and Emotional Assessment Program (LEAP) at Massachusetts General Hospital and Assistant Professor of Psychology at Harvard Medical School. The coauthor of *Straight Talk about Psychological Testing for Kids*, Dr. Braaten lives with her family in Boston.

Brian Willoughby, PhD, is Staff Psychologist at LEAP and a faculty member at Harvard Medical School. Dr. Willoughby specializes in neuropsychological assessments of children and adolescents with learning, developmental, and emotional concerns. He is married and lives in Boston.